Table of Content

Table of Content 1
Chapter 1: Introduction 3
Chapter 2: Safety and Precautions 14
Chapter 3: Carrier Oils and Emulsifiers 23
Chapter 4: Inhalation Techniques 32
Chapter 5: Topical Applications 39
Chapter 6: Aromatherapy for Common Ailments 48
Chapter 7: Aromatherapy for Specific Conditions 61
Chapter 8: Aromatherapy for Women's Health 76
Chapter 9: Aromatherapy for Children 85
Chapter 10: Aromatherapy for the Elderly 94
Chapter 11: Advanced Aromatherapy Techniques 104
Chapter 12: Real-World Case Studies 112
Chapter 13: Business and Practice Considerations 121
Chapter 14: Continuing Education and Certification 130
Chapter 15: Research and Evidence 137
Chapter 16: Quality and Regulation 145
Chapter 17: Plant Profiles 153
Chapter 18: Blending Formulations..................................... 159

Chapter 19: Resources 166
Chapter 20: Conclusion 175

Chapter 1: Introduction

The History and Science of Aromatherapy

The Greeks and Romans also embraced aromatherapy, with Hippocrates, the father of medicine, advocating the use of aromatic plants for their healing properties. Dioscorides, a Greek physician and botanist, compiled a comprehensive Materia Medica in the first century AD, which included detailed descriptions of over 600 medicinal plants, many of which were used for aromatherapy.

In the Middle Ages, aromatherapy flourished in the Arab world. Arabian physicians, such as Avicenna, developed sophisticated methods for extracting and distilling essential oils. They also introduced the use of aromatherapy for psychological and emotional well-being.

During the Renaissance, aromatherapy experienced a revival in Europe, with physicians and alchemists experimenting with the therapeutic applications of essential oils. Paracelsus, a Swiss physician and alchemist, coined the term "aromatherapy" in the 16th century, referring to the use of aromatic substances for medicinal purposes.

The modern era of aromatherapy began in the early 20th century with the work of French chemist René-Maurice Gattefossé. Gattefossé accidentally burned his hand in his laboratory and instinctively plunged it into a vat of lavender oil. To his astonishment, the burn healed quickly and without scarring. This incident sparked Gattefossé's interest in the therapeutic properties of essential oils, and he devoted the rest of his life to studying and promoting aromatherapy.

The Science Behind Aromatherapy

Aromatherapy works by stimulating the olfactory system, which is responsible for our sense of smell. When we inhale essential oils, the aromatic molecules travel through the nasal passages and bind to receptors in the olfactory bulb. These receptors then send signals to the brain, where they can trigger a variety of physiological and psychological responses.

Essential oils are complex mixtures of hundreds of different compounds, each with its own unique therapeutic properties. Some of the most common and well-studied essential oils include lavender, peppermint, eucalyptus, and tea tree oil.

Lavender oil is known for its calming and relaxing effects. It has been shown to reduce anxiety, promote sleep, and alleviate pain. Peppermint oil is invigorating and stimulating. It can help to improve focus, reduce headaches, and relieve nausea. Eucalyptus oil is decongestant and antiseptic. It can help to clear congestion, boost immunity, and relieve respiratory problems. Tea tree oil is antimicrobial and antifungal. It can help to fight infections, treat acne, and promote wound healing.

The Therapeutic Benefits of Aromatherapy

Aromatherapy has been shown to provide a wide range of therapeutic benefits, both physical and emotional. Some of the most well-documented benefits include:

Stress and anxiety relief: Essential oils such as lavender, chamomile, and bergamot have been shown to reduce stress and anxiety levels.
Improved sleep: Essential oils such as lavender, valerian, and ylang-ylang can help to promote relaxation and improve sleep quality.
Pain relief: Essential oils such as peppermint, eucalyptus, and rosemary have analgesic properties and can help to relieve pain from headaches, muscle aches, and sprains.
Enhanced mood: Essential oils such as citrus oils, jasmine, and rose can help to uplift mood and combat depression.
Boosted immunity: Essential oils such as eucalyptus, tea tree oil, and oregano have antimicrobial and antiviral properties and can help to boost immunity.
Skincare: Essential oils such as lavender, tea tree oil, and frankincense have antibacterial and anti-inflammatory properties and can help to improve skin health.

How to Use Aromatherapy

Aromatherapy can be enjoyed in a variety of ways, including:

Inhalation: Inhaling essential oils through a diffuser, humidifier, or personal inhaler is a simple and effective way to experience their therapeutic benefits.
Topical application: Essential oils can be diluted with a carrier oil, such as jojoba or coconut oil, and applied to the skin for massage, baths, or compresses.
Oral ingestion: Some essential oils are safe to ingest in small amounts, but this should only be done under the guidance of a qualified healthcare professional.

Safety Considerations

Essential oils are concentrated plant extracts and should be used with care. Some essential oils can cause skin irritation or allergic reactions, especially when applied undiluted. It is always best to do a patch test on a small area of skin before using any essential oil.

Some essential oils are toxic if ingested and should never be taken orally without the guidance of a qualified healthcare professional. These include essential oils such as pennyroyal, thuja, and wormwood.

Essential oils should also be used with caution during pregnancy and by people with certain medical conditions. It is always best to consult with a qualified healthcare professional before using essential oils if you have any concerns.

Aromatherapy is a safe and effective way to improve your physical, emotional, and mental well-being. Its rich history and proven therapeutic benefits make it a valuable tool for health and healing. By using essential oils wisely, you can harness the power of nature to promote relaxation, reduce stress, relieve pain, boost immunity, and enhance your overall quality of life.

Essential Oil Chemistry

Classification and Structure

Essential oils are primarily composed of terpenes and terpenoids, hydrocarbons characterized by their isoprene units. Terpenes consist of two or more isoprene units linked together, while terpenoids contain oxygenated derivatives of terpenes. These compounds can be classified based on their structure:

Monoterpenes: Two isoprene units, often found in citrus fruits (e. g. , limonene, pinene)
Sesquiterpenes: Three isoprene units, frequently encountered in herbs and spices (e. g. , caryophyllene, humulene)
Diterpenes: Four isoprene units, present in resins and woods (e. g. , camphor, abietic acid)

Functional Groups

The biological activity of essential oils is largely determined by the presence of functional groups. These groups interact with biological molecules, influencing the oil's therapeutic effects:

Alcohols: Hydroxyl group (-OH), contributing to

antibacterial and antiviral properties (e. g. , geraniol, linalool)
Aldehydes: Carbonyl group (-CHO), often responsible for stimulating effects (e. g. , citral, cinnamaldehyde)
Esters: Carboxylic acid and alcohol group (-COO-), imparting calming and sedative properties (e. g. , linalyl acetate, geranyl acetate)
Ketones: Carbonyl group between two carbon atoms (-CO-), often found in antiseptic and anti-inflammatory oils (e. g. , camphor, carvone)
Phenols: Hydroxyl group attached to an aromatic ring (-OH), exhibiting strong antibacterial and antiviral activity (e. g. , thymol, carvacrol)

Extraction and Analysis

Essential oils are extracted from plant material through various methods, including:

Steam distillation: Plant material is heated with steam, releasing volatile compounds.
Hydrodistillation: Plant material is immersed in water and boiled, vaporizing the essential oils.
Cold pressing: Essential oils are extracted from the peel of citrus fruits.

Gas chromatography-mass spectrometry (GC-MS) is the primary technique used to analyze essential oils. This method separates and identifies individual compounds based on their volatility and mass-to-charge ratio.

Therapeutic Properties

The therapeutic properties of essential oils are attributed to their chemical composition:

Antimicrobial: Some essential oils, such as tea tree oil and oregano oil, possess strong antibacterial, antifungal, and antiviral activity.
Anti-inflammatory: Essential oils containing terpenes and terpenoids, such as eucalyptus and rosemary, have been shown to reduce inflammation.
Anxiolytic: Oils like lavender and chamomile contain linalool and other esters that promote relaxation and reduce anxiety.
Antioxidant: Essential oils rich in phenolic compounds, such as clove and cinnamon, exhibit antioxidant activity, protecting cells from damage.

Safety Considerations

While essential oils offer numerous health benefits, it's important to use them safely:

Skin sensitivity: Some essential oils can cause skin irritation or allergic reactions.
Internal use: Essential oils should not be ingested unless under the guidance of a qualified healthcare professional.
Drug interactions: Certain essential oils may interact with medications.
Pregnancy and lactation: Some essential oils are contraindicated during pregnancy or lactation.

Understanding the chemistry of essential oils is essential

for appreciating their therapeutic potential and safe use. Their complex composition of terpenes, terpenoids, and functional groups underlies their wide range of therapeutic properties. By adhering to safety guidelines, individuals can harness the healing benefits of essential oils to enhance their well-being.

Therapeutic Uses of Aromatherapy

Essential oils are highly concentrated plant extracts obtained through various methods such as steam distillation, cold pressing, or solvent extraction. They contain a complex blend of volatile compounds, including terpenes, alcohols, esters, and ketones, which impart their characteristic aromas and therapeutic properties. Aromatherapy involves inhaling or applying essential oils topically to promote relaxation, alleviate stress, and address a wide range of physical and emotional ailments.

Stress and Anxiety Relief:

Stress and anxiety are prevalent issues in modern society, and aromatherapy offers a natural approach to calming the mind and promoting relaxation. Essential oils like lavender, chamomile, and bergamot have sedative and anxiolytic effects, reducing feelings of stress, tension, and nervousness. Inhaling these oils through a diffuser or applying them topically in diluted form can help slow down the heart rate, lower blood pressure, and induce a sense of tranquility.

Sleep Improvement:

Sleep disturbances are a common problem that can significantly impact overall health and well-being. Certain essential oils, such as lavender, chamomile, and vetiver, possess calming and sleep-promoting properties. By creating a relaxing atmosphere at bedtime, aromatherapy can help reduce sleep latency, improve sleep quality, and enhance overall sleep duration.

Pain Management:

Aromatherapy has been used for centuries to alleviate pain. Essential oils like peppermint, eucalyptus, and rosemary have analgesic and anti-inflammatory properties. When applied topically or inhaled, these oils can provide temporary relief from headaches, muscle pain, and joint pain. The cooling and stimulating effects of these oils can help reduce inflammation and improve blood circulation, promoting pain relief.

Skin Care:

Essential oils have a wide range of applications in skincare due to their antimicrobial, antioxidant, and anti-inflammatory properties. Tea tree oil, known for its antiseptic qualities, is commonly used to treat acne, wounds, and skin infections. Lavender and chamomile oils possess calming and soothing effects, making them beneficial for reducing skin irritation, redness, and inflammation. Additionally, essential oils like frankincense and myrrh promote skin regeneration and reduce the appearance of wrinkles and fine lines.

Respiratory Support:

Essential oils like eucalyptus, peppermint, and rosemary have expectorant and decongestant properties. When inhaled through a diffuser or steam inhalation, these oils can help clear nasal congestion, reduce inflammation in the airways, and promote easier breathing. Aromatherapy can be particularly beneficial for individuals with respiratory conditions such as asthma, bronchitis, and the common cold.

Digestive Health:

Certain essential oils, including peppermint, ginger, and fennel, have digestive benefits. Inhaling or ingesting these oils can help relieve symptoms of indigestion, gas, and bloating. They can stimulate digestive enzymes, promote bile production, and improve overall gut health.

Emotional Well-being:

Aromatherapy has been used for centuries to promote emotional well-being and balance. Essential oils like rose, jasmine, and ylang-ylang have uplifting and euphoric effects, helping to reduce feelings of sadness, depression, and anxiety. They can stimulate the release of endorphins, promote positive emotions, and enhance self-esteem.

Precautions:

While aromatherapy is generally considered safe, it is important to use essential oils with caution and under the guidance of a qualified healthcare professional. Some essential oils can cause skin irritation or allergic reactions, particularly when used undiluted. It is crucial to dilute essential oils in a carrier oil, such as jojoba, almond, or coconut oil, before applying them topically.

Individuals with certain health conditions, pregnant women, and young children should exercise extra caution when using essential oils. It is always advisable to consult with a healthcare provider before incorporating aromatherapy into your health routine. From stress relief and sleep improvement to pain management, skin care, and respiratory support, aromatherapy offers a wide range of therapeutic benefits. However, it is essential to use essential oils safely and under the guidance of a qualified healthcare professional to maximize their benefits and minimize any potential risks.

Chapter 2: Safety and Precautions

Essential Oil Safety Guidelines

Understanding Essential Oil Potency and Toxicity

Essential oils are highly concentrated and can be toxic if ingested or used undiluted on the skin. Different oils possess varying levels of potency, and some may be more sensitizing or irritating than others. It is essential to research the specific oil you intend to use and understand its potential side effects before incorporating it into your routine.

Proper Dilution for Safe Use

To ensure safety, essential oils should always be diluted in a carrier substance before topical application. Carrier substances, such as vegetable oils (e. g. , jojoba, coconut, or almond oil), help dilute the potency of essential oils and reduce the risk of skin irritation. The recommended dilution ratio varies depending on the oil and intended use, typically ranging from 2-5% for most applications.

Skin Sensitivity Testing

Before using any essential oil topically, it is advisable to perform a skin sensitivity test. Dilute the oil as recommended and apply a small amount to a patch of skin on the inner forearm. Observe the area for any signs of irritation, redness, or discomfort for 24-48 hours. If any adverse reaction occurs, discontinue use and consult a healthcare professional.

Avoid Internal Use

Essential oils are not meant for internal consumption, and ingesting them can be extremely dangerous. Some oils, such as camphor and wintergreen, contain toxic compounds that can cause severe health issues, including liver damage and seizures. Only consume essential oils under the direct supervision of a qualified healthcare practitioner.

Inhalation Safety

Inhaling essential oils can be beneficial for respiratory conditions, but caution is still necessary. Avoid excessive inhalation, as some oils can irritate the mucous membranes. Use a diffuser sparingly, and always ensure proper ventilation when using essential oils in enclosed spaces.

Pregnancy and Children

Certain essential oils may be contraindicated for use during pregnancy or on children. Some oils can cause uterine contractions or may be harmful to developing organs. Consult with a healthcare professional before using essential oils if you are pregnant, breastfeeding, or have children.

Storage and Handling

Store essential oils in dark glass bottles away from direct sunlight and heat. Exposure to light and high temperatures can degrade the oil's constituents and reduce their effectiveness. Keep oils out of reach of children and pets, and handle them with care to prevent spills and accidents.

Respecting Essential Oil Limits

Avoid using essential oils excessively or for prolonged periods. Each oil has recommended daily and weekly limits, which should not be exceeded to prevent potential health risks. Refer to reputable sources or consult a healthcare practitioner for specific usage guidelines.

Seek Professional Advice When Needed

If you have any concerns or underlying health conditions, it is highly recommended to consult with a qualified healthcare practitioner before using essential oils. They can provide personalized guidance and ensure safe and appropriate use based on your individual needs.

Essential oils can be powerful allies for health and well-being when used safely and responsibly. By adhering to these guidelines, you can harness the benefits of these natural substances while minimizing risks. Remember to dilute properly, perform skin sensitivity tests, avoid internal use, and seek professional advice when needed. With knowledge and caution, essential oils can be a valuable addition to your holistic health toolkit.

Contraindications and Cautions

Absolute Contraindications

Absolute contraindications are conditions that make exercise unsafe under any circumstances. These conditions include:

Unstable angina
Myocardial infarction (heart attack)
Severe aortic stenosis
Dissecting aortic aneurysm
Pulmonary embolism
Deep vein thrombosis
Uncontrolled hypertension
Severe heart failure
Recent stroke
Transient ischemic attack (TIA)
Uncontrolled seizures
Severe mental illness
Pregnancy with certain complications

Relative Contraindications

Relative contraindications are conditions that may make exercise inadvisable in some cases, but not in others.

These conditions include:

Stable angina
Mild aortic stenosis
Mild heart failure
Controlled hypertension
Mild arrhythmias
Diabetes
Obesity
Osteoporosis
Arthritis
Chronic obstructive pulmonary disease (COPD)
Asthma
Sickle cell anemia

If you have any of these conditions, it is important to talk to your doctor before starting an exercise program. Your doctor can help you determine if it is safe for you to exercise and, if so, what type of exercise is best for you.

Cautions for Exercise

Even if you do not have any contraindications to exercise, there are some precautions you should take to avoid injury. These precautions include:

Start slowly and gradually increase the intensity and duration of your workouts.
Listen to your body and stop if you experience any pain.
Warm up before each workout and cool down afterwards.
Stay hydrated by drinking plenty of fluids before, during, and after your workouts.
Wear appropriate clothing and footwear.

Exercise in a safe environment.

If you have any questions or concerns about exercise, be sure to talk to your doctor.

Here are some additional tips for exercising safely if you have a chronic condition:

Work with your doctor to develop an exercise plan that is safe and effective for you.
Start slowly and gradually increase the intensity and duration of your workouts.
Listen to your body and stop if you experience any pain.
Warm up before each workout and cool down afterwards.
Stay hydrated by drinking plenty of fluids before, during, and after your workouts.
Wear appropriate clothing and footwear.
Exercise in a safe environment.
Be aware of your symptoms and stop exercising if they worsen.

By following these tips, you can help reduce your risk of injury and make exercise a safe and enjoyable part of your life.

Blending and Formulating Safely

Understanding Essential Oil Properties

Essential oils are highly concentrated plant extracts that possess potent therapeutic properties. Each essential oil has unique chemical constituents that determine its specific aroma, therapeutic benefits, and potential hazards.

Before blending or formulating with essential oils, it's essential to research and understand their individual properties. Reliable sources, such as reputable books, articles, or consultations with qualified aromatherapists, can provide valuable information on the therapeutic uses, contraindications, and safety precautions for each essential oil.

Safe Blending Practices

When blending essential oils, it's crucial to consider their compatibility and potential interactions. Avoid combining oils that are known to have adverse reactions with each other. For example, peppermint oil should not be blended with homeopathic remedies as it can interfere with their effectiveness. Additionally, certain essential oils, such as cinnamon bark and oregano, are considered "hot oils" and should be used sparingly in blends to prevent skin irritation.

Appropriate Dilution

Essential oils are highly concentrated and can be irritating to the skin if used undiluted. It's essential to dilute essential oils in a carrier substance, such as a vegetable oil (e. g. , jojoba, almond, or coconut oil) or unscented lotion, before applying them topically. The recommended dilution ratio varies depending on the intended use and the sensitivity of the individual's skin. For topical applications, a dilution of 2-5% is generally safe for most adults. However, it's advisable to start with a lower dilution and gradually increase the concentration as tolerated.

Safe Formulation Techniques

When formulating essential oil blends, it's important to consider the purpose of the blend and the desired therapeutic outcome. Different essential oils possess complementary properties that can enhance each other's effects. For example, blending lavender oil with chamomile oil can create a calming and relaxing blend, while combining rosemary oil with peppermint oil can stimulate circulation and improve focus. Experiment with different combinations to find the blend that best suits your needs.

Storage and Handling Precautions

Proper storage and handling of essential oils are crucial for maintaining their therapeutic properties and ensuring safety. Essential oils should be stored in dark glass bottles away from direct sunlight and heat. Avoid storing them in plastic containers as they may react with the oils. Always keep essential oils out of reach of children and pets. When handling essential oils, avoid direct contact with the skin or eyes. If contact occurs, dilute the oil with a carrier substance and rinse the affected area thoroughly with water.

Blending and formulating essential oils safely requires a comprehensive understanding of their properties, potential hazards, and appropriate handling techniques. By adhering to these guidelines, you can create safe and effective essential oil blends that enhance your well-being and promote a healthy lifestyle. Remember to prioritize safety by researching the properties of essential oils, diluting them appropriately, and storing them properly. With knowledge and responsible use, essential oils can become valuable tools for holistic health and well-being.

Chapter 3: Carrier Oils and Emulsifiers

Choosing and Using Carrier Oils

Factors to Consider When Choosing a Carrier Oil

Skin Type: Different carrier oils have varying properties that suit different skin types. For example, jojoba oil is ideal for oily or acne-prone skin due to its non-comedogenic nature, while avocado oil is rich in nutrients that nourish dry or aging skin.
Absorption Rate: The absorption rate of a carrier oil influences how quickly essential oils penetrate the skin. Lighter oils like grapeseed oil absorb rapidly, providing immediate benefits, while heavier oils like castor oil have a slower absorption rate and offer sustained effects.
Viscosity: Viscosity refers to the thickness or flowability of a carrier oil. Thicker oils like coconut oil create a protective barrier on the skin, while thinner oils like almond oil spread easily and are suitable for massage.
Aroma: Some carrier oils have distinct aromas that may complement or interfere with the scents of essential oils. Neutral-scented oils like fractionated coconut oil or grapeseed oil are preferred for blends where the

therapeutic properties of essential oils are the primary focus.
Shelf Life: The shelf life of a carrier oil is influenced by its fatty acid composition. Oils rich in saturated fats, like coconut oil, have a longer shelf life than those high in unsaturated fats, like sunflower oil.

Common Carrier Oils and Their Properties

Jojoba Oil: Non-comedogenic, similar to sebum, suitable for oily and acne-prone skin.
Avocado Oil: Rich in vitamins and antioxidants, nourishing for dry and aging skin.
Grapeseed Oil: Light, rapidly absorbed, neutral aroma, ideal for massage blends.
Almond Oil: Light, hypoallergenic, suitable for sensitive skin.
Fractionated Coconut Oil: Liquid at room temperature, odorless, long shelf life, good carrier for essential oils.
Olive Oil: Rich in antioxidants, protective and moisturizing for the skin.
Castor Oil: Thick, slow-absorbing, emollient and anti-inflammatory properties.

Guidelines for Using Carrier Oils

Dilution Ratios: The recommended dilution ratio for essential oils varies depending on the intended use and the potency of the oil. For topical application, a 2-5% dilution is generally considered safe. This translates to 10-25 drops of essential oil per ounce of carrier oil.
Storage: Carrier oils should be stored in dark, cool places away from direct sunlight and heat. This helps preserve

their shelf life and prevent oxidation.
Allergy Testing: Before using any new carrier oil, perform a patch test on a small area of skin to ensure there are no allergic reactions.
Avoid Contamination: Always use clean equipment and containers when handling carrier oils and essential oils to prevent contamination.
Internal Use: Some carrier oils, such as coconut oil, are suitable for internal use, while others are not. Always consult with a qualified healthcare professional before ingesting carrier oils.

Choosing and using carrier oils is an essential aspect of aromatherapy and essential oil blending. By considering the factors discussed above, you can select the most appropriate carrier oil for your individual needs and enhance the therapeutic benefits of your essential oil blends. Remember to follow the guidelines for dilution, storage, and usage to ensure the safe and effective application of carrier oils.

Emulsifiers for Water-Based Blends

The hydrophilic portion of the emulsifier molecule interacts strongly with water molecules, forming a protective layer around the oil droplets. This layer prevents the droplets from coalescing, which would lead to phase separation. The hydrophobic portion, on the other hand, interacts with the oil molecules, ensuring their dispersion throughout the aqueous phase.

The effectiveness of an emulsifier is primarily determined by its hydrophilic-lipophilic balance (HLB). HLB is a numerical scale that quantifies the relative strength of the hydrophilic and hydrophobic regions of the emulsifier. An emulsifier with a high HLB value (above 10) is more water-soluble and suitable for stabilizing oil-in-water (O. W) emulsions, where oil droplets are dispersed in a continuous water phase. Conversely, emulsifiers with a low HLB value (below 10) are more oil-soluble and effective in stabilizing water-in-oil (W. O) emulsions, where water droplets are dispersed in a continuous oil phase.

Types of Emulsifiers

The realm of emulsifiers encompasses a vast array of compounds, each tailored to specific applications and desired properties. Some of the most commonly used emulsifiers include:

Ionic emulsifiers: These emulsifiers possess a net electrical charge, which enhances their interaction with water molecules. They are particularly effective in stabilizing emulsions containing high concentrations of electrolytes.

Nonionic emulsifiers: These emulsifiers lack a net electrical charge, making them versatile and compatible with a wide range of ingredients. They are often used in food, cosmetic, and pharmaceutical formulations.

Natural emulsifiers: These emulsifiers are derived from natural sources, such as plants and animals. Examples include lecithin (from egg yolks) and gum arabic (from acacia trees).

Applications of Emulsifiers in Water-Based Blends

Emulsifiers play a crucial role in a multitude of water-based blends, including:

Food products: Emulsifiers enhance the texture, stability, and shelf life of food products such as mayonnaise, salad dressings, ice cream, and baked goods.

Cosmetics: Emulsifiers are responsible for the smooth, creamy texture of lotions, creams, and shampoos. They also help to stabilize fragrances and prevent phase separation.

Pharmaceuticals: Emulsifiers are used to enhance the bioavailability and stability of drugs by facilitating their dispersion in aqueous solutions.

Industrial products: Emulsifiers are employed in various industrial applications, such as the production of paints, coatings, and lubricants.

Selection of Emulsifiers for Water-Based Blends

The selection of an appropriate emulsifier for a water-based blend depends on several factors, including:

Nature of the oil and water phases: The HLB value of the emulsifier should match the polarity of the oil and water phases.

Desired emulsion type (O. W or W. O): The HLB value of

the emulsifier determines the type of emulsion that will be formed.

Concentration of electrolytes: Ionic emulsifiers may be more suitable for blends with high electrolyte concentrations.

Compatibility with other ingredients: The emulsifier should be compatible with all other ingredients in the blend, including active ingredients, fragrances, and preservatives.

Emulsifiers are indispensable components of water-based blends, ensuring their stability, homogeneity, and desired properties. By carefully selecting the appropriate emulsifier based on the specific requirements of the blend, formulators can create stable and effective products that meet the demands of consumers and industries alike.

Creams and Lotions for Topical Use

Creams: Thick, Emollient, and Occlusive

Creams are thick, semi-solid formulations that contain a high oil content. They provide a protective layer on the skin, reducing water loss and preventing dehydration. Creams are ideal for dry, flaky, or irritated skin. They are commonly used to treat conditions like eczema, psoriasis, and diaper rash.

The emollient properties of creams make them effective in softening the skin and reducing itching. The occlusive nature of creams helps retain moisture and prevents external irritants from penetrating the skin. However, creams can sometimes feel greasy and may not be suitable for oily or acne-prone skin.

Lotions: Liquid, Lighter, and Refreshing

Lotions are liquid or semi-liquid formulations that contain a lower oil content compared to creams. They are lighter and less greasy, making them a more suitable option for oily or sensitive skin. Lotions are easily spreadable and absorbed, providing a cooling and refreshing sensation.

Due to their lower oil content, lotions do not provide the same level of emolliency and occlusion as creams. They are primarily used to hydrate the skin and prevent dryness. Lotions are commonly used for daily skin care routines, sun protection, and mild skin irritations.

Choosing the Right Formulation

The choice between a cream or lotion depends on the specific skin condition and individual preferences. Here are some guidelines to consider:

Dry, irritated, or inflamed skin: Creams are better suited for these conditions as they provide a thicker protective layer and intense moisturization.
Oily or sensitive skin: Lotions are a better option for these skin types as they are lighter, less greasy, and less likely to clog pores.
Daily skin care: Lotions are a good choice for daily use to keep the skin hydrated and protected.

Sun protection: Lotions can be formulated with sunscreen ingredients, providing both hydration and sun protection in one convenient product.

Specific skin conditions: Some skin conditions may require specific formulations designed to address their unique needs. Consult a healthcare professional for personalized recommendations.

Common Ingredients in Creams and Lotions

Both creams and lotions contain a variety of ingredients to achieve their desired effects. Some common ingredients include:

Emollients: These ingredients, such as petrolatum, lanolin, and mineral oil, soften and smooth the skin, reducing dryness and flakiness.

Occlusives: These ingredients, such as beeswax and silicones, form a protective barrier on the skin, preventing water loss and protecting from external irritants.

Humectants: These ingredients, such as glycerin and hyaluronic acid, attract and retain water in the skin, providing deep hydration.

Active ingredients: Depending on the intended purpose, creams and lotions may contain specific active ingredients, such as antibiotics, anti-inflammatories, or anti-itching agents, to address underlying skin conditions.

Safe and Effective Use of Creams and Lotions

To ensure safe and effective use of creams and lotions, follow these guidelines:

Read the label carefully: Pay attention to the ingredients, directions for use, and any precautions.

Start with a small amount: Apply a small amount to a test patch of skin first to check for any reactions.

Apply as directed: Follow the application instructions provided on the product label.

Avoid excessive use: Using too much cream or lotion can clog pores or irritate the skin.

Store properly: Keep creams and lotions in a cool, dry place, away from heat and light.

Discard expired products: Replace old creams and lotions with fresh ones to maintain their effectiveness.

By understanding the differences between creams and lotions and choosing the right formulation for your skin, you can effectively address various skin conditions and maintain healthy, radiant skin.

Chapter 4: Inhalation Techniques

Direct Inhalation (Diffusers and Nebulizers)

Diffusers

Diffusers are devices that disperse essential oils into the air. They do this by using a fan or a heat source to create a fine mist that can be inhaled. Diffusers are a popular way to use essential oils because they are easy to use and can be used in any room.

There are two main types of diffusers: ultrasonic diffusers and nebulizing diffusers. Ultrasonic diffusers use high-frequency sound waves to create a fine mist, while nebulizing diffusers use a high-pressure air stream to create a fine mist.

Ultrasonic diffusers are less expensive than nebulizing diffusers, but they can be noisier. Nebulizing diffusers are more expensive than ultrasonic diffusers, but they are quieter and produce a finer mist.

Nebulizers

Nebulizers are devices that convert liquid medication into a fine mist that can be inhaled. Nebulizers are often used to deliver medications to people with respiratory conditions, such as asthma and chronic obstructive pulmonary disease (COPD).

There are two main types of nebulizers: jet nebulizers and ultrasonic nebulizers. Jet nebulizers use a high-pressure air stream to create a fine mist, while ultrasonic nebulizers use high-frequency sound waves to create a fine mist.

Jet nebulizers are less expensive than ultrasonic nebulizers, but they can be noisier. Ultrasonic nebulizers are more expensive than jet nebulizers, but they are quieter and produce a finer mist.

Benefits of Direct Inhalation

Direct inhalation is a safe and effective way to deliver essential oils and other therapeutic substances to the lungs. Direct inhalation can provide a number of benefits, including:

Improved respiratory health
Reduced stress and anxiety
Improved sleep
Boosted immunity
Reduced pain
Improved skin health

Safety Considerations

Direct inhalation is generally safe, but there are a few safety considerations to keep in mind.

Do not use essential oils that are not intended for inhalation. Some essential oils can be toxic if inhaled. Do not use diffusers or nebulizers for more than 30 minutes at a time. This can lead to respiratory irritation. Keep diffusers and nebulizers out of reach of children and pets.
If you have any respiratory conditions, talk to your doctor before using diffusers or nebulizers.

Direct inhalation is a safe and effective way to deliver essential oils and other therapeutic substances to the lungs. Direct inhalation can provide a number of benefits, including improved respiratory health, reduced stress and anxiety, improved sleep, boosted immunity, reduced pain, and improved skin health.

Indirect Inhalation (Steam Inhalation and Compresses)

Steam inhalation can be done using a variety of methods. One common method is to boil water in a pot and then place the pot on a table or counter. Cover your head with a towel and inhale the steam for 10-12 minutes. You can also use a commercial steam inhaler, which is a device that produces steam from a heated water reservoir.

Steam inhalation is generally safe for most people.

However, it is important to take precautions to avoid burns. Do not place your face too close to the steam, and do not inhale the steam for more than 12 minutes at a time. If you have any concerns about steam inhalation, talk to your doctor.

Compresses

Compresses are another common home remedy for nasal congestion and other respiratory problems. They involve applying a warm or cold compress to the affected area. Warm compresses help to increase blood flow and reduce inflammation. Cold compresses help to numb the pain and reduce swelling.

Compresses can be made using a variety of materials, such as towels, washcloths, or gauze. To make a warm compress, soak a cloth in warm water and then wring it out. To make a cold compress, soak a cloth in cold water and then wring it out.

Apply the compress to the affected area for 10-15 minutes. You can repeat the process several times a day. Compresses are generally safe for most people. However, it is important to take precautions to avoid burns or frostbite. Do not apply a warm compress to an open wound, and do not apply a cold compress for more than 15 minutes at a time. If you have any concerns about using compresses, talk to your doctor.

Benefits of Indirect Inhalation and Compresses

Indirect inhalation and compresses can provide a number

of benefits for people with nasal congestion and other respiratory problems. These benefits include:

Thinning mucus and making it easier to expel
Relieving inflammation
Opening up the airways
Reducing pain and swelling
Improving sleep quality

Indirect inhalation and compresses are safe and effective home remedies that can help to relieve nasal congestion and other respiratory problems. If you are experiencing these problems, talk to your doctor about whether indirect inhalation or compresses may be right for you.

Aromatic Baths

Origins and Ancient Rituals

The origins of aromatic baths can be traced back to ancient civilizations, with references found in Egyptian, Greek, and Roman texts. Egyptians believed that bathing in fragrant oils and herbs purified the body and spirit, while the Greeks associated aromatic baths with relaxation and rejuvenation. The Romans, known for their elaborate bathing rituals, constructed opulent bathhouses where citizens could indulge in therapeutic and social bathing.

Therapeutic Benefits of Essential Oils

The therapeutic benefits of aromatic baths stem from the essential oils released from aromatic plants and herbs. These oils contain volatile compounds that are absorbed through the skin or inhaled, providing both physical and emotional effects.

Pain Relief and Relaxation: Essential oils such as lavender, chamomile, and eucalyptus have analgesic and anti-inflammatory properties, making them effective for reducing pain and promoting relaxation.
Improved Sleep: Inhaling the calming scents of essential oils like lavender and valerian root can induce relaxation and improve sleep quality.
Respiratory Support: Eucalyptus, rosemary, and pine essential oils have expectorant and decongestant properties, making them beneficial for clearing respiratory congestion.
Emotional Well-being: Essential oils like bergamot, frankincense, and ylang-ylang have mood-boosting and calming effects, promoting emotional balance and reducing stress.

Creating an Aromatic Bath Experience

Creating an aromatic bath experience at home is simple and enjoyable. Here are some tips:

Choose Essential Oils: Select essential oils based on your desired therapeutic effects. Consider a blend of oils to enhance the overall experience.
Prepare the Bath: Fill the bathtub with warm water and add 5-10 drops of essential oils per gallon of water. Stir gently to disperse the oils.
Relax and Soak: Submerge yourself in the aromatic bath for 15-20 minutes, allowing the oils to work their magic.
Enhance the Experience: Dim the lights, play soothing

music, or add candles for a relaxing ambiance.

Precautions and Considerations

Skin Sensitivity: Some essential oils may cause skin irritation in sensitive individuals. Perform a patch test on a small area of skin before using them in the bath.
Pregnancy and Nursing: Certain essential oils may be harmful to pregnant or nursing women. Consult a healthcare professional before using aromatic baths during these periods.
Dosage: Use essential oils in moderation. Excessive use can overwhelm the senses and cause adverse effects.
Interactions: Some essential oils may interact with certain medications. Consult a doctor or pharmacist if you have any concerns.

Aromatic baths offer a unique and therapeutic way to care for both your physical and mental well-being. By harnessing the power of essential oils, you can transform your bathroom into a sanctuary for relaxation, rejuvenation, and healing. Whether you seek pain relief, improved sleep, or emotional balance, an aromatic bath is a time-honored tradition that can enhance your overall health and well-being.

Chapter 5: Topical Applications

Massage and Blending for Topical Use

There are many different types of massage, each with its own unique benefits. Some of the most common types of massage include:

Swedish massage: This is a gentle, relaxing massage that uses long, flowing strokes to promote relaxation and relieve tension.
Deep tissue massage: This is a more intense massage that uses deep pressure to release chronic muscle tension and knots.
Sports massage: This type of massage is designed to help athletes prepare for and recover from athletic activity. It can help to improve flexibility, reduce muscle soreness, and prevent injuries.
Prenatal massage: This type of massage is designed for pregnant women. It can help to relieve pregnancy-related aches and pains, and promote relaxation.
Infant massage: This type of massage is designed for infants. It can help to promote bonding between parent and child, and relieve gas and colic.

Massage has been shown to have a number of benefits, including:

Reduces stress and anxiety: Massage can help to reduce levels of stress hormones, such as cortisol, and promote relaxation.
Relieves pain: Massage can help to relieve pain from a variety of sources, including muscle tension, headaches, and back pain.
Improves circulation: Massage can help to improve circulation by increasing blood flow to the massaged area.
Increases flexibility: Massage can help to increase flexibility by stretching muscles and connective tissues.
Promotes relaxation: Massage can help to promote relaxation by reducing muscle tension and promoting a sense of calm.

Blending for Topical Use

Blending essential oils for topical use is a great way to create custom blends that can be used for a variety of purposes, such as pain relief, relaxation, and skin care. When blending essential oils, it is important to use high-quality oils and to follow proper dilution guidelines.

To make a topical blend, you will need the following:

Essential oils of your choice
Carrier oil, such as jojoba oil, coconut oil, or almond oil
A glass bottle or jar
A dropper

To make a topical blend, follow these steps:

1. Choose the essential oils you want to use. You can use a single oil or a blend of oils.
2. Add the essential oils to the glass bottle or jar.
3. Add the carrier oil to the bottle or jar. The amount of carrier oil you need will depend on the desired dilution.
4. Shake the bottle or jar well to combine the oils.
5. Apply the blend to the desired area of skin.

When blending essential oils for topical use, it is important to follow proper dilution guidelines. This will help to prevent skin irritation and other adverse reactions. The recommended dilution for topical use is 2-5% essential oils in a carrier oil.

Safety Considerations

When using massage or essential oils, it is important to take the following safety considerations into account:

Do not use massage or essential oils on open wounds or irritated skin.
Do not use essential oils on children under the age of 6.
Do not use essential oils during pregnancy or breastfeeding.
Do not use essential oils if you have any known allergies.
If you have any concerns, talk to your doctor before using massage or essential oils.

Massage and blending essential oils for topical use are two

great ways to improve your health and well-being. Massage can help to reduce stress, relieve pain, and improve flexibility. Blending essential oils for topical use can help to create custom blends that can be used for a variety of purposes, such as pain relief, relaxation, and skin care. When using massage or essential oils, it is important to follow proper safety guidelines to ensure your safety.

Essential Oils for Skin Care

Understanding Essential Oils

Essential oils are hydrophobic, meaning they repel water. This property allows them to penetrate the skin's lipid barrier, delivering their therapeutic constituents directly to the underlying tissues. Essential oils are highly concentrated, so it is crucial to dilute them with a carrier oil, such as jojoba or almond oil, before topical application. The recommended dilution ratio for skincare is typically 2-3 drops of essential oil per 10ml of carrier oil.

Choosing the Right Essential Oils for Your Skin Type

The choice of essential oils for skincare depends on your skin type and the specific concerns you wish to address. Here are some general guidelines:

Dry skin: Lavender, chamomile, and rosehip essential oils are known for their hydrating and soothing properties.
Oily skin: Tea tree, rosemary, and lemon essential oils can help regulate sebum production and reduce inflammation.
Sensitive skin: Chamomile, lavender, and calendula essential oils are gentle and calming, minimizing irritation.

Mature skin: Frankincense, myrrh, and rose essential oils promote cell regeneration and reduce the appearance of fine lines and wrinkles.
Acne-prone skin: Tea tree, lavender, and rosemary essential oils possess antibacterial and anti-inflammatory properties, helping to clear and prevent breakouts.

Incorporating Essential Oils into Your Skincare Routine

Essential oils can be incorporated into your skincare routine in various ways:

Facial cleansing: Add a few drops of essential oils to your regular cleanser or create a gentle cleansing blend with a carrier oil.
Toning: Dilute essential oils with water to create a refreshing and balancing facial toner.
Moisturizing: Add a few drops of essential oils to your favorite moisturizer or create your own custom blend using a carrier oil.
Facial masks: Combine essential oils with natural ingredients, such as clay or honey, to create nourishing and targeted facial masks.
Steam facials: Add a few drops of essential oils to a bowl of hot water and inhale the aromatic steam to promote circulation and detoxification.

Safety Considerations

While essential oils are generally safe for topical use, certain precautions should be taken:

Always dilute essential oils with a carrier oil before applying

them to the skin.
Perform a patch test on a small area of skin to check for any allergic reactions.
Avoid using essential oils on broken or irritated skin. Some essential oils, such as citrus oils, can cause photosensitivity, so it is best to avoid sun exposure after application.
If you are pregnant or breastfeeding, consult with a qualified healthcare professional before using essential oils.

Essential oils offer a wide range of benefits for skin health, providing a natural and effective way to address various concerns. By understanding the different essential oils and their properties, and by following the safety guidelines, you can harness their power to achieve healthy, radiant skin. Essential oils are a valuable addition to any holistic skincare routine, promoting both the external beauty and well-being of your skin.

Essential Oils for Hair Care

The Science of Essential Oils for Hair

Essential oils exert their effects on hair through various mechanisms. They contain a complex array of volatile compounds that interact with the hair shaft and scalp environment. Some essential oils possess antibacterial and antifungal properties, helping to combat scalp infections and promote a healthy scalp microbiome. Others contain antioxidants that protect against damage caused by environmental stressors, such as UV radiation and pollution.

Benefits of Essential Oils for Hair

Incorporating essential oils into your hair care routine can offer a multitude of benefits, including:

Promoting hair growth: Certain essential oils, such as rosemary and lavender, have been shown to stimulate hair follicles and promote hair growth.
Reducing hair loss: Essential oils like peppermint and tea tree oil may help to reduce hair loss by addressing underlying scalp issues, such as dandruff and inflammation.
Improving hair strength and texture: Essential oils rich in vitamins and minerals, such as jojoba oil and argan oil, can nourish and strengthen hair, improving its texture and elasticity.
Treating scalp conditions: Essential oils with antibacterial and antifungal properties, such as tea tree oil and lavender oil, can help to alleviate scalp conditions such as dandruff, psoriasis, and eczema.
Balancing scalp pH: Essential oils like lemon oil and ylang-ylang oil can help to balance the pH level of the scalp, creating an optimal environment for healthy hair growth.

Applications of Essential Oils for Hair

Essential oils can be incorporated into your hair care routine in various ways:

Shampoo: Add a few drops of essential oil to your

shampoo and massage it into the scalp and hair. Leave it in for a few minutes before rinsing.
Conditioner: Mix a few drops of essential oil into your conditioner and apply it to the hair, focusing on the ends. Leave it in for a few minutes before rinsing.
Scalp massage oil: Dilute a few drops of essential oil in a carrier oil, such as jojoba oil or coconut oil. Massage the mixture into the scalp for several minutes. Leave it in for at least 30 minutes before washing.
Hair rinse: Add a few drops of essential oil to a cup of water and pour it over the hair after washing. Do not rinse.

Safe Usage Practices

When using essential oils for hair care, it is important to follow safe usage practices:

Dilution: Always dilute essential oils in a carrier oil before applying them to the hair or scalp. This helps to prevent skin irritation and sensitization.
Skin test: Before using an essential oil on your hair, perform a skin patch test on a small area of your skin to rule out any allergic reactions.
Avoid sun exposure: Some essential oils, such as citrus oils, can cause photosensitivity. Avoid applying them to the hair before sun exposure.
Storage: Store essential oils in a cool, dark place away from children and pets.

Essential oils offer a wealth of benefits for hair health, promoting hair growth, reducing hair loss, improving hair strength and texture, treating scalp conditions, and balancing scalp pH. By incorporating these potent botanical extracts into your hair care routine, you can harness the power of nature to achieve healthy, beautiful hair. Always remember to dilute essential oils and perform a skin patch test before use, and consult with a qualified healthcare professional for any specific hair concerns.

Chapter 6: Aromatherapy for Common Ailments

Respiratory Conditions

Types of Respiratory Conditions

1. Asthma: A chronic inflammatory condition characterized by recurring episodes of wheezing, coughing, chest tightness, and shortness of breath. It is triggered by various factors such as allergens, exercise, cold air, and stress.

2. Chronic Obstructive Pulmonary Disease (COPD): A group of progressive lung diseases that cause airflow limitation, including chronic bronchitis and emphysema. COPD is primarily caused by smoking and long-term exposure to harmful particles.

3. Pneumonia: An infection of the lungs caused by bacteria, viruses, or fungi. It can range from mild to severe, leading to fever, cough, shortness of breath, and chest pain.

4. Acute Bronchitis: An inflammation of the bronchi, the main airways leading to the lungs. It is usually caused by a viral infection and results in cough, chest congestion, and fever.

5. Tuberculosis (TB): A bacterial infection that primarily affects the lungs. It can spread through close contact with an infected person and cause symptoms such as cough, weight loss, and fatigue.

6. Lung Cancer: A malignant tumor that develops in the lungs. It is the leading cause of cancer-related deaths worldwide and is primarily caused by smoking.

7. Cystic Fibrosis: An inherited condition that affects the lungs, pancreas, and other organs. It causes thick, sticky mucus to accumulate in the airways, leading to breathing difficulties, infections, and digestive issues.

Causes of Respiratory Conditions

1. Smoking: One of the leading causes of respiratory conditions, especially COPD and lung cancer. Smoking damages the airways and lungs, leading to inflammation and scarring.

2. Air Pollution: Exposure to particulate matter, ozone, and other air pollutants can irritate the respiratory system, triggering asthma attacks and worsening COPD.

3. Infections: Respiratory infections, such as pneumonia and bronchitis, are caused by bacteria, viruses, or fungi

that enter the airways and cause inflammation and infection.

4. Allergens: Allergens such as pollen, dust mites, and pet dander can trigger asthma and allergic rhinitis, leading to respiratory symptoms like wheezing and sneezing.

5. Genetics: Some respiratory conditions, such as cystic fibrosis and certain types of lung cancer, are caused by genetic mutations that affect the function of the respiratory system.

Symptoms of Respiratory Conditions

The symptoms of respiratory conditions vary depending on the underlying cause and severity. Common symptoms include:

1. Coughing

2. Shortness of breath

3. Wheezing

4. Chest pain

5. Chest congestion

6. Fever

7. Fatigue

8. Weight loss

Treatment Options for Respiratory Conditions

Treatment for respiratory conditions aims to alleviate symptoms, prevent complications, and improve overall lung function. Treatment options may include:

1. Medications: Inhalers, nebulizers, and oral medications are used to reduce inflammation, open airways, and fight infections.

2. Oxygen Therapy: Supplemental oxygen is provided to increase the oxygen levels in the blood for individuals with severe respiratory conditions.

3. Surgery: In some cases, surgery may be necessary to remove lung tumors, repair damaged airways, or treat certain lung diseases.

4. Lifestyle Modifications: Quitting smoking, avoiding air pollutants, and managing allergies can significantly improve respiratory health.

5. Pulmonary Rehabilitation: A supervised program that includes exercise, education, and support to help individuals with respiratory conditions improve their breathing and overall well-being.

Respiratory conditions are a diverse group of ailments that can significantly impact an individual's quality of life. Understanding the different types of respiratory conditions, their causes, symptoms, and treatment options is crucial for effective management and prevention. By taking proactive steps to reduce risk factors, seeking timely medical attention, and adhering to recommended treatment plans, individuals can improve their respiratory health and maintain optimal lung function.

Digestive Issues

Gastroesophageal reflux disease (GERD) is a condition in which stomach acid flows back into the esophagus. This can cause heartburn, chest pain, and difficulty swallowing. Peptic ulcer disease is a condition in which sores develop in the lining of the stomach or small intestine. This can cause pain, bleeding, and vomiting.
Irritable bowel syndrome (IBS) is a condition that causes abdominal pain, cramping, and diarrhea or constipation. Inflammatory bowel disease (IBD) is a condition that causes chronic inflammation of the digestive tract. This can lead to abdominal pain, diarrhea, weight loss, and fatigue. Diverticular disease is a condition in which small pouches form in the walls of the colon. These pouches can become infected or inflamed, causing pain, bleeding, and constipation.

Digestive issues can be caused by a variety of factors, including:

Diet
Stress
Medications
Medical conditions
Genetics

In most cases, digestive issues can be managed with lifestyle changes, such as:

Eating a healthy diet
Getting regular exercise
Managing stress
Avoiding smoking and alcohol

If lifestyle changes do not improve your symptoms, your doctor may recommend medication or surgery.

Diet

The foods you eat can have a significant impact on your digestive health. Eating a healthy diet can help to prevent and relieve digestive issues. A healthy diet for digestive health includes:

Plenty of fruits and vegetables. Fruits and vegetables are high in fiber, which is essential for good digestive health. Fiber helps to keep your bowels moving and prevents constipation.
Whole grains. Whole grains are also a good source of fiber. They are also a good source of complex carbohydrates, which provide energy and help to keep you feeling full.
Lean protein. Lean protein is a good source of amino acids, which are essential for building and repairing tissues.
Low-fat dairy products. Low-fat dairy products are a good source of calcium, which is essential for strong bones.
Healthy fats. Healthy fats, such as those found in olive oil

and avocados, can help to reduce inflammation and improve digestive health.

Stress

Stress can trigger or worsen digestive issues. When you are stressed, your body releases hormones that can slow down digestion and cause stomach pain and diarrhea. To manage stress, try:

Exercise
Yoga
Meditation
Spending time in nature
Talking to a therapist

Medications

Some medications can cause digestive side effects, such as:

Nonsteroidal anti-inflammatory drugs (NSAIDs), such as ibuprofen and naproxen, can cause stomach pain, bleeding, and ulcers.
Aspirin can cause stomach pain and bleeding.
Steroids can cause stomach pain, bleeding, and ulcers.
Chemotherapy drugs can cause nausea, vomiting, and diarrhea.

If you are taking any medications that are causing digestive side effects, talk to your doctor about ways to reduce these side effects.

Medical conditions

Some medical conditions can cause digestive issues, such as:

Diabetes can cause gastroparesis, a condition in which the stomach empties slowly. This can lead to nausea, vomiting, and abdominal pain.
Thyroid disease can cause constipation or diarrhea.
Celiac disease is a condition in which the body cannot tolerate gluten, a protein found in wheat, rye, and barley. This can lead to abdominal pain, diarrhea, and weight loss.
Crohn's disease and ulcerative colitis are types of inflammatory bowel disease that can cause abdominal pain, diarrhea, and weight loss.

If you have a medical condition that is causing digestive issues, your doctor will recommend treatment for the underlying condition.

Genetics

Some people are more likely to develop digestive issues due to their genes. For example, people with a family history of peptic ulcer disease are more likely to develop the condition themselves.

If you have a family history of digestive issues, talk to your doctor about ways to reduce your risk of developing these conditions.

Musculoskeletal Pain

Causes of Musculoskeletal Pain

The origins of musculoskeletal pain are multifaceted, often stemming from various factors. Physical exertion, repetitive motions, poor posture, and injuries are common triggers. Age-related degeneration, such as osteoarthritis, can also contribute to the development of pain. Certain medical conditions, including fibromyalgia and rheumatoid arthritis, can also manifest as musculoskeletal discomfort. Additionally, psychological factors, such as stress and anxiety, have been linked to the perception and exacerbation of pain.

Treatment Options for Musculoskeletal Pain

Addressing musculoskeletal pain requires a tailored approach that considers the underlying cause, severity, and individual circumstances. A range of treatment options is available, including:

Medications: Over-the-counter pain relievers, such as ibuprofen and acetaminophen, can provide temporary relief. Prescription medications, including opioids and muscle relaxants, may be necessary for more severe pain.
Physical Therapy: Physical therapists utilize exercises, stretches, and manual techniques to restore range of motion, reduce pain, and improve muscle function.
Occupational Therapy: Occupational therapists focus on adapting daily activities and modifying workspaces to minimize pain and maximize functionality.
Alternative Therapies: Acupuncture, massage therapy, and chiropractic care have shown promise in alleviating musculoskeletal pain.

Surgery: In rare cases, surgery may be necessary to correct structural abnormalities or repair damaged tissues.

Preventing Musculoskeletal Pain

Proactive measures can significantly reduce the risk of developing musculoskeletal pain or minimize its recurrence. Here are some preventive strategies:

Maintaining good posture: Correct posture while sitting, standing, and sleeping helps distribute weight evenly and reduces strain on muscles and joints.
Engaging in regular exercise: Regular physical activity strengthens muscles, improves flexibility, and promotes overall well-being.
Using proper lifting techniques: Avoid lifting heavy objects with improper form, which can strain muscles and cause injury.
Taking breaks: Regular breaks during prolonged activities or repetitive motions can prevent muscle fatigue and reduce the risk of pain.
Managing stress: Stress can exacerbate pain perception. Engaging in stress-reducing activities, such as yoga or meditation, can help mitigate its impact.

Musculoskeletal pain is a common condition with various causes and treatment options. Understanding the underlying mechanisms and exploring available therapies can empower individuals to effectively manage their pain. By adopting preventive measures, such as maintaining good posture, exercising regularly, and managing stress, individuals can minimize the risk of developing or recurring musculoskeletal pain and enjoy an active and fulfilling life.

Stress and Emotional Well-being

Stress arises from various sources, including environmental stressors (e. g. , work demands, financial burdens), life events (e. g. , divorce, bereavement), and internal stressors (e. g. , negative thoughts, anxiety). When we encounter stressors, our bodies activate the "fight-or-flight" response, releasing hormones such as cortisol and adrenaline. This response increases heart rate, blood pressure, and muscle tension, preparing us for action or withdrawal.

However, chronic or severe stress can lead to the dysregulation of the stress response system, resulting in a persistent state of high arousal and physiological strain. This can manifest in a range of physical and mental health problems, including anxiety disorders, depression, heart disease, and diabetes.

Impact of Stress on Emotional Well-being

Stress profoundly influences our emotional well-being, affecting our mood, thoughts, and behaviors. Chronic stress can lead to:

Emotional Exhaustion: Persistent stress depletes our emotional resources, leaving us feeling drained, apathetic, and unable to cope with everyday challenges.

Anxiety: Stress can trigger excessive worry, nervousness, and feelings of unease. It can disrupt sleep, impair concentration, and make it difficult to function effectively.

Depression: Chronic stress increases the risk of developing depression, characterized by persistent sadness, loss of interest in activities, and feelings of worthlessness and hopelessness.

Mood Swings: Stress can cause fluctuations in mood, leading to irritability, anger, or tearfulness. It can disrupt relationships and impair social functioning.

Cognitive Impairment: Stress can impair cognitive function, affecting memory, attention, and problem-solving abilities. It can hinder our ability to think clearly and make sound decisions.

Strategies for Managing Stress and Promoting Emotional Well-being

Recognizing the negative impact of stress on our emotional well-being, it is crucial to develop effective coping strategies to manage stress and promote emotional health. Here are some evidence-based strategies:

Identify Stressors: The first step to managing stress is to identify the sources of stress in our lives. By pinpointing the stressors, we can develop targeted strategies to address them.

Cognitive Restructuring: This technique involves challenging negative thoughts and replacing them with more positive and realistic ones. By reframing our thoughts, we can reduce stress and improve our emotional outlook.

Mindfulness: Mindfulness practices, such as meditation and deep breathing exercises, help us cultivate present-moment awareness and reduce stress. By focusing on the present, we can let go of worries about the future or regrets about the past.

Physical Activity: Exercise is a powerful stress reliever. Regular physical activity releases endorphins, which have mood-boosting effects. It also improves sleep and cardiovascular health, contributing to overall well-being.

Social Support: Connecting with loved ones and maintaining a strong social network can provide emotional support and reduce stress. Talking to others about our problems, seeking advice, and sharing experiences can alleviate our burden and enhance our emotional resilience.

Self-Care: Prioritizing self-care is essential for managing stress and promoting emotional well-being. This includes getting enough sleep, eating a healthy diet, and engaging in activities that bring joy and relaxation.

Professional Help: If stress becomes overwhelming and interferes with our daily functioning, it is important to seek professional help. Therapy can provide a safe and supportive environment to explore the causes of stress, develop coping mechanisms, and improve emotional well-being.

Chapter 7: Aromatherapy for Specific Conditions

Anxiety and Depression

The Diagnostic and Statistical Manual of Mental Disorders (DSM-5) classifies anxiety disorders into several categories, each with distinct symptoms and characteristics:

- Generalized anxiety disorder (GAD): Persistent, excessive worry about a variety of topics, accompanied by physical symptoms like restlessness, fatigue, and muscle tension.
- Panic disorder: Recurrent, unexpected panic attacks characterized by intense fear, shortness of breath, heart palpitations, and dizziness.
- Phobias: Intense, irrational fears of specific objects, situations, or activities, such as social interactions (social phobia) or heights (acrophobia).
- Social anxiety disorder (SAD): Excessive fear or anxiety in social situations, leading to avoidance and significant distress.
- Obsessive-compulsive disorder (OCD): Persistent,

intrusive thoughts (obsessions) that trigger repetitive behaviors (compulsions), such as excessive hand washing or checking.

Anxiety disorders often arise from a complex interplay of genetic, psychological, and environmental factors. They can be triggered by life events, such as trauma, loss, or major life changes, or by underlying medical conditions, substance use, or certain medications.

Symptoms and Consequences of Anxiety

The symptoms of anxiety can vary depending on the specific disorder and individual, but common manifestations include:

- Excessive worry and rumination
- Physical symptoms: rapid heart rate, sweating, trembling, muscle tension
- Restlessness and agitation
- Difficulty concentrating and making decisions
- Irritability and mood swings
- Sleep problems
- Avoidance of feared situations or activities

Untreated anxiety can have significant consequences for individuals' personal, academic, and professional lives. It can lead to social isolation, impaired academic performance, occupational difficulties, and diminished overall well-being. Anxiety disorders are also associated with an increased risk of other mental health conditions, such as depression.

Depression: The Shadow of Despair

Depression is a serious mood disorder characterized by persistent feelings of sadness, emptiness, and loss of interest in activities that once brought joy. It is often accompanied by physical, cognitive, and behavioral symptoms that interfere with everyday functioning.

According to the DSM-5, depression is diagnosed when an individual experiences at least five of the following symptoms for a period of two weeks or more:

- Depressed mood most of the day, nearly every day
- Loss of interest or pleasure in activities that were once enjoyable
- Significant weight loss or gain (not due to dieting) or changes in appetite
- Insomnia or hypersomnia (excessive sleeping)
- Fatigue or loss of energy
- Feelings of worthlessness or excessive guilt
- Difficulty concentrating or making decisions
- Recurrent thoughts of death or suicide

Depression can result from a combination of biological, psychological, and social factors. It can be triggered by life events, such as the loss of a loved one or a major setback, or by underlying medical conditions, substance use, or certain medications.

Symptoms and Consequences of Depression

The symptoms of depression can range in severity from mild to severe and can include:

- Persistent sadness, hopelessness, and emptiness
- Loss of interest in activities that once brought pleasure
- Changes in appetite and weight
- Sleep disturbances
- Fatigue and loss of energy
- Irritability and mood swings
- Difficulty concentrating and making decisions
- Feelings of worthlessness or guilt
- Suicidal thoughts or behaviors

Untreated depression can have devastating consequences for individuals and their loved ones. It can lead to social isolation, impaired academic performance, occupational difficulties, and diminished overall well-being. Depression is also associated with an increased risk of physical health problems, such as heart disease, stroke, and diabetes.

Comorbidity of Anxiety and Depression

Anxiety and depression frequently co-occur, with up to 60% of individuals with anxiety disorders also experiencing depression, and vice versa. This comorbidity can complicate diagnosis and treatment, as symptoms of one disorder may overlap with those of the other.

The co-occurrence of anxiety and depression is thought to be related to shared underlying mechanisms, such as neurotransmitter imbalances, genetic factors, and environmental stressors. Additionally, anxiety can trigger depressive symptoms, while depression can worsen anxiety symptoms, creating a vicious cycle.

Treatment Options for Anxiety and Depression

Fortunately, effective treatments are available for anxiety and depression. These treatments may include:

- Psychotherapy: Cognitive-behavioral therapy (CBT), exposure and response prevention (ERP), and interpersonal therapy (IPT) are evidence-based psychotherapies that have been shown to effectively reduce symptoms of anxiety and depression.
- Medication: Antidepressants, such as selective serotonin reuptake inhibitors (SSRIs) and serotonin-norepinephrine reuptake inhibitors (SNRIs), can help to regulate neurotransmitter imbalances and alleviate symptoms of depression. Anti-anxiety medications, such as benzodiazepines and buspirone, can provide short-term relief from anxiety symptoms.
- Lifestyle changes: Regular exercise, healthy sleep habits, stress management techniques, and a balanced diet can support overall mental health and well-being.
- Complementary therapies: Some individuals may find relief from anxiety and depression through complementary therapies, such as mindfulness-based stress reduction (MBSR), acupuncture, or massage therapy.

Overcoming Anxiety and Depression: A Path to Recovery

Overcoming anxiety and depression is a challenging but achievable goal. With proper diagnosis, treatment, and support, individuals can manage their symptoms and reclaim their quality of life. It is important to remember that anxiety and depression are common and treatable conditions, and that seeking help is a sign of strength and resilience. By confronting these challenges head-on, individuals can embark on a path to recovery and build a brighter future.

Chronic Pain

Chronic pain encompasses a diverse spectrum of conditions, ranging from musculoskeletal disorders like osteoarthritis and fibromyalgia to neuropathic pain caused by nerve damage and cancer pain. Its etiology is often complex and multifactorial, involving a combination of physical, psychological, and social factors. While tissue injury may trigger chronic pain, it is not always the primary cause. In many cases, the underlying mechanisms are poorly understood, making diagnosis and treatment challenging.

Understanding the Complexities of Chronic Pain

Chronic pain is not merely a physical sensation; it is a complex interplay of physiological, psychological, and social factors. The physiological mechanisms underlying chronic pain involve alterations in the nervous system, leading to heightened sensitivity to pain and an amplification of pain signals. This phenomenon, known as central sensitization, results in a state of chronic pain that is disproportionate to the actual tissue damage.

The psychological and social dimensions of chronic pain are equally significant. Patients with chronic pain often experience anxiety, depression, and sleep disturbances. They may withdraw from social activities, leading to isolation and diminished quality of life. The stigma associated with chronic pain can further compound their suffering, as they may be perceived as exaggerating or malingering.

Managing Chronic Pain: An Interdisciplinary Approach

Effectively managing chronic pain requires a comprehensive and interdisciplinary approach that addresses both the physical and psychological aspects of the condition. Treatment strategies may include a combination of pharmacological interventions, physical and occupational therapy, psychological counseling, and lifestyle modifications.

Pharmacological interventions commonly involve the use of non-steroidal anti-inflammatory drugs (NSAIDs), opioids, and other pain medications. However, these medications often provide only partial relief and can have significant side effects. Physical and occupational therapy can help improve range of motion, reduce muscle spasms, and enhance functional capacity.

Psychological counseling, including cognitive-behavioral therapy (CBT) and acceptance and commitment therapy (ACT), can help patients develop coping mechanisms, manage stress, and reduce the psychological impact of chronic pain. Mindfulness-based interventions have also shown promise in improving pain perception and reducing psychological distress.

Lifestyle modifications, such as regular exercise, weight loss, and smoking cessation, can positively impact chronic pain. Exercise releases endorphins, which have pain-relieving effects, and can strengthen muscles and improve overall health. Weight loss can reduce pressure on joints and improve mobility. Quitting smoking can improve circulation and reduce inflammation.

Advances in Chronic Pain Research

Research into chronic pain is ongoing, with significant advancements being made in understanding the mechanisms of pain and developing new treatment approaches. One promising area is the use of targeted therapies, such as monoclonal antibodies and gene therapy, to modulate specific pathways involved in chronic pain.

Another area of focus is the development of personalized medicine for chronic pain. By considering individual genetic and epigenetic factors, researchers aim to tailor treatments to each patient's unique needs, improving efficacy and reducing side effects. While there is no universal cure, effective management strategies exist that can significantly reduce pain levels, improve function, and enhance quality of life. An interdisciplinary approach that addresses the physical, psychological, and social aspects of chronic pain is essential for successful outcomes. Continued research holds promise for further advancements in understanding and treating chronic pain, offering hope to those who suffer from this relentless condition.

Insomnia

Causes of Insomnia

The causes of insomnia are multifaceted and can be broadly categorized into two main types: primary and secondary.

Primary insomnia is a standalone condition that is not directly caused by any underlying medical or psychological issues. It can be triggered by factors such as stress, anxiety, or changes in circadian rhythm.
Secondary insomnia is a symptom of another underlying medical or psychological condition. These conditions can include depression, anxiety disorders, chronic pain, and endocrine disorders.

Symptoms of Insomnia

The primary symptom of insomnia is difficulty falling or staying asleep. Other symptoms may include:

Waking up frequently during the night
Feeling tired or unrested during the day
Difficulty concentrating
Irritability
Memory problems

Consequences of Insomnia

Chronic insomnia can have significant consequences on an individual's physical, mental, and emotional health. These consequences include:

Physical health: Increased risk of cardiovascular disease,

obesity, and diabetes
Mental health: Exacerbation of anxiety and depression, increased risk of suicidal thoughts and behaviors
Emotional well-being: Fatigue, irritability, difficulty regulating emotions

Treatment Options

The treatment of insomnia depends on the underlying cause and severity of the condition. Common treatment options include:

Behavioral therapy: Techniques such as cognitive behavioral therapy for insomnia (CBT-I) help individuals identify and change negative thoughts and behaviors that contribute to insomnia.
Medication: Prescription sleep aids, such as benzodiazepines and non-benzodiazepine hypnotics, can provide short-term relief from insomnia symptoms. However, they should be used cautiously due to the potential for side effects and dependency.
Lifestyle modifications: Establishing regular sleep-wake cycles, creating a relaxing bedtime routine, and avoiding caffeine and alcohol before bed can improve sleep quality.
Other therapies: Acupuncture, massage therapy, and yoga have shown promising results in reducing insomnia symptoms.

Seeking Professional Help

If insomnia persists despite self-help measures, it is recommended to seek professional help. A healthcare professional can assess the underlying cause of the insomnia and recommend the most appropriate treatment plan.

Insomnia is a common and potentially debilitating sleep disorder that can have significant consequences on an individual's health and well-being. Understanding the causes, symptoms, and treatment options for insomnia is essential for effective management of the condition. By addressing the underlying causes and implementing appropriate treatment strategies, individuals can improve their sleep quality and enhance their overall health and well-being.

Autoimmune Disorders

Autoimmune disorders can affect any part of the body, including the skin, joints, muscles, nervous system, and organs. Symptoms of autoimmune disorders vary depending on the specific disorder, but they may include fatigue, pain, swelling, stiffness, rash, and organ damage.

There are more than 100 different autoimmune disorders, and the exact cause of most of them is unknown. However, it is thought that autoimmune disorders are caused by a combination of genetic and environmental factors.

Risk Factors for Autoimmune Disorders

Anyone can develop an autoimmune disorder, but certain factors may increase the risk, including:

Family history: People who have a family history of autoimmune disorders are more likely to develop one themselves.
Gender: Women are more likely to develop autoimmune disorders than men.
Age: Autoimmune disorders can develop at any age, but they are most common in people between the ages of 20 and 40.
Certain infections: Some infections may trigger autoimmune disorders.
Environmental factors: Exposure to certain chemicals, toxins, and pollutants may increase the risk of autoimmune disorders.

Symptoms of Autoimmune Disorders

Symptoms of autoimmune disorders vary depending on the specific disorder. However, some common symptoms include:

Fatigue
Pain
Swelling
Stiffness
Rash
Organ damage

Diagnosis of Autoimmune Disorders

Diagnosing an autoimmune disorder can be challenging. There is no single test that can diagnose all autoimmune disorders. Doctors typically diagnose autoimmune disorders based on a patient's symptoms, a physical examination, and blood tests. Blood tests can detect antibodies that are produced by the immune system to attack the body's own tissues.

Treatment of Autoimmune Disorders

There is no cure for autoimmune disorders. However, there are treatments that can help to manage symptoms and prevent organ damage. Treatment options for autoimmune disorders include:

Medications: Medications can be used to suppress the immune system and reduce inflammation.
Lifestyle changes: Lifestyle changes, such as diet and exercise, can help to improve symptoms and overall health.
Surgery: Surgery may be necessary to treat organ damage caused by autoimmune disorders.

Outlook for Autoimmune Disorders

The outlook for people with autoimmune disorders varies depending on the specific disorder. Some autoimmune disorders are mild and can be managed with medication and lifestyle changes. Others are more serious and can lead to significant disability and organ damage.

Prevention of Autoimmune Disorders

There is no sure way to prevent autoimmune disorders. However, there are some things that people can do to reduce their risk, including:

Eating a healthy diet: Eating a healthy diet can help to

boost the immune system and reduce inflammation.
Getting regular exercise: Regular exercise can help to improve overall health and reduce stress.
Avoiding exposure to toxins: Avoiding exposure to certain chemicals, toxins, and pollutants can help to reduce the risk of autoimmune disorders.
Managing stress: Stress can trigger autoimmune disorders. Managing stress can help to reduce the risk of developing an autoimmune disorder.

Living with an Autoimmune Disorder

Living with an autoimmune disorder can be challenging. However, there are things that people can do to cope with the challenges and live a full and productive life. These include:

Educating yourself about your disorder: Learning about your disorder can help you to better understand your symptoms and treatment options.
Joining a support group: Joining a support group can provide you with emotional support and information from others who are living with autoimmune disorders.
Taking care of your mental health: Autoimmune disorders can take a toll on your mental health. It is important to take care of your mental health by talking to a therapist or counselor.
Living a healthy lifestyle: Eating a healthy diet, getting regular exercise, and managing stress can help to improve your overall health and well-being.

Autoimmune disorders are a serious concern, but they can be managed with proper treatment and lifestyle changes.

By educating yourself about your disorder and taking care of your physical and mental health, you can live a full and productive life.

Chapter 8: Aromatherapy for Women's Health

Menstrual Cramps and Irregularities

The exact cause of menstrual cramps is not fully understood, but it is believed to be related to the levels of prostaglandins in the body. Prostaglandins are hormone-like substances that cause the uterus to contract. Higher levels of prostaglandins can lead to more intense cramps.

There are a number of things that can be done to relieve menstrual cramps. Some simple measures include:

Applying heat to the lower abdomen
Taking over-the-counter pain relievers, such as ibuprofen or naproxen
Getting regular exercise
Eating a healthy diet
Getting enough sleep

In some cases, more severe cramps may require

prescription medication or even surgery.

Irregular Periods: Causes and Concerns

Irregular periods are another common problem that many women experience. Irregular periods can be caused by a variety of factors, including:

Hormonal imbalances
Thyroid problems
Polycystic ovary syndrome (PCOS)
Pregnancy
Breastfeeding
Certain medications
Stress

Irregular periods can be a sign of an underlying health condition, so it is important to see a doctor if you are experiencing this problem.

There are a number of things that can be done to regulate irregular periods, including:

Lifestyle changes, such as losing weight, eating a healthy diet, and getting regular exercise
Hormonal therapy
Surgery

When to See a Doctor

It is important to see a doctor if you are experiencing severe menstrual cramps or irregular periods. This is especially important if you are also experiencing other symptoms, such as:

Heavy bleeding
Pain that is not relieved by over-the-counter pain relievers
Fever
Chills
Nausea and vomiting

These symptoms could be a sign of an underlying health condition that requires treatment.

Menstrual cramps and irregular periods are common problems that many women experience. While these problems can be uncomfortable and disruptive, there are a number of things that can be done to relieve the symptoms and improve your quality of life. If you are experiencing severe menstrual cramps or irregular periods, it is important to see a doctor to rule out any underlying health conditions.

Pregnancy and Childbirth

From the moment of conception, a complex symphony of hormonal signals initiates a cascade of biological events. The fertilized egg implants in the uterine lining, where it undergoes rapid cell division to form an embryo. As the embryo develops, it becomes enveloped in a protective membrane and amniotic fluid, forming the amniotic sac. By the end of the first trimester, the major organs and systems of the fetus have begun to form, and the heart begins to beat.

Throughout the pregnancy, the mother's body undergoes significant adaptations to support the growing fetus. The uterus expands dramatically, accommodating the growing baby. The placenta, a specialized organ that connects the mother's blood supply to the fetus, develops and facilitates the exchange of nutrients and waste products. The mother's blood volume increases to meet the increased metabolic demands of pregnancy.

Hormonal changes play a crucial role in pregnancy. Estrogen and progesterone, the primary hormones involved, promote the growth of the uterus and breasts. They also suppress uterine contractions and relax the muscles of the cervix. Other hormones, such as prolactin, prepare the breasts for lactation.

Childbirth: The Culmination of Pregnancy

Childbirth, also known as labor and delivery, is the physiological process by which the fetus is expelled from the uterus. It is a complex and often intense experience that typically involves three stages.

Stage 1: Labor

Labor begins with regular, rhythmic contractions of the uterus. These contractions gradually increase in frequency and intensity, causing the cervix to dilate (open). As the cervix dilates, the baby's head begins to descend into the birth canal. This stage can last several hours or even days.

Stage 2: Delivery

Once the cervix is fully dilated, the second stage of labor begins. The mother typically experiences strong, involuntary urges to push. With each contraction, the baby is gradually pushed down the birth canal and eventually emerges from the vagina. This stage typically lasts a few minutes to an hour.

Stage 3: Placental Delivery

After the baby is born, the third stage of labor involves the delivery of the placenta. The placenta typically separates from the uterine wall within a few minutes of the baby's birth. The mother may be asked to push or cough to help expel the placenta.

Postpartum Period: Recovery and Adjustment

After childbirth, the mother enters the postpartum period, which typically lasts six to eight weeks. During this time, her body undergoes a gradual return to its pre-pregnancy state. The uterus contracts to shrink back to its original size, and the hormones that supported pregnancy gradually decline. The mother may experience vaginal bleeding, breast tenderness, and other physical changes.

Emotionally, the postpartum period can be a time of both joy and adjustment. The mother may experience a range of emotions, including happiness, exhaustion, anxiety, and baby blues (a temporary period of sadness). With time and support, most mothers adapt to the challenges and rewards of parenthood.

Prenatal Care: Ensuring a Healthy Pregnancy

Prenatal care is essential for promoting a healthy pregnancy and ensuring the well-being of both the mother and baby. Regular prenatal visits with a healthcare provider allow for:

Monitoring the mother's and baby's health
Identifying and managing any potential risks
Providing education and support on pregnancy, labor, and delivery
Screening for genetic disorders and other health conditions

Prenatal care also includes healthy lifestyle habits, such as eating a nutritious diet, exercising regularly, and avoiding harmful substances like alcohol and tobacco. By following prenatal care recommendations, women can significantly improve the chances of having a safe and healthy pregnancy.

Pregnancy and childbirth are transformative experiences that encompass profound physical, emotional, and social changes. With proper prenatal care and support, women can navigate these experiences with confidence and ensure the well-being of their babies. Understanding the physiological processes involved in pregnancy and childbirth empowers expectant mothers to make informed decisions and advocate for their own health and the health of their children.

Menopause

Physiological Changes during Menopause

Menopause is triggered by a decline in the production of estrogen and progesterone hormones by the ovaries. These hormonal changes lead to a range of physical symptoms, including:

Hot flashes: Sudden feelings of intense heat and sweating
Night sweats: Profuse sweating during sleep
Sleep disturbances: Difficulty falling or staying asleep
Mood swings: Irritability, anxiety, or depression
Vaginal dryness and atrophy: Thinning and inflammation of the vaginal walls
Loss of bone density: Increased risk of osteoporosis
Changes in body weight and composition: Redistribution of body fat

Psychological and Emotional Aspects of Menopause

Menopause can also have a significant impact on a woman's psychological and emotional well-being. It can be a time of both liberation and loss, as women come to terms with the end of their reproductive abilities and the aging process.

Common emotional experiences during menopause include:

Grief or sadness over the loss of fertility
Anxiety about physical changes and health risks
Concerns about body image and attractiveness

Feelings of liberation from the constraints of menstruation
A sense of empowerment and newfound purpose

Managing Menopause Symptoms

While menopause is a natural process, its symptoms can be disruptive and uncomfortable. Fortunately, there are a range of treatment options available to alleviate symptoms and improve overall well-being.

Hormone replacement therapy (HRT): HRT replaces the declining levels of estrogen and progesterone to alleviate hot flashes, night sweats, and vaginal dryness.
Selective estrogen receptor modulators (SERMs): These medications have similar effects to HRT but may have a lower risk of side effects.
Antidepressants: Certain antidepressants can help reduce hot flashes and mood swings.
Lifestyle modifications: Exercise, a healthy diet, and stress management techniques can all help improve symptoms and overall well-being during menopause.

Long-Term Health Implications of Menopause

The hormonal changes of menopause increase a woman's risk of developing certain health conditions, including:

Osteoporosis: Loss of bone density can lead to increased risk of fractures.
Cardiovascular disease: Declining estrogen levels may contribute to a higher risk of heart disease and stroke.
Cognitive decline: Some studies suggest that menopause may be associated with an increased risk of cognitive

impairment.

Navigating Menopause with Support

Menopause is a significant life event that can bring both challenges and opportunities for growth. Having a support system in place can help women navigate this transition with greater ease.

Medical professionals: Doctors and other healthcare providers can provide medical advice, support, and treatment options.
Therapists or counselors: Talking to a therapist can help women process the emotional and psychological aspects of menopause.
Family and friends: Sharing experiences and seeking support from loved ones can provide comfort and understanding.
Support groups: Connecting with other women going through similar experiences can offer valuable camaraderie and emotional support.

Menopause is a natural and inevitable part of a woman's life. While it can bring about a range of physical and emotional changes, it is important to remember that it is not a disease or a sign of decline. With proper management of symptoms and a supportive network, women can navigate menopause with confidence and continue to live fulfilling and meaningful lives.

Chapter 9: Aromatherapy for Children

Safe Essential Oils for Children

Safety Considerations

The safety of essential oils for children depends on several factors:

Concentration: Essential oils are highly concentrated and should always be diluted before use. Improper dilution can lead to skin irritation or other adverse reactions.
Age: The age of the child is crucial in determining which oils are appropriate and at what concentration. Certain oils may not be suitable for younger children.
Individual Sensitivity: Children may exhibit different sensitivities to essential oils, even if they are generally considered safe. It is essential to observe your child closely for any signs of irritation or allergic reactions.
Medical Conditions: Children with specific medical conditions may need to avoid certain essential oils or use

them only under the guidance of a healthcare professional.

Appropriate Essential Oils for Children

When selecting essential oils for children, opt for those that are gentle and specifically formulated for their delicate skin and systems. Some commonly used safe essential oils for children include:

Lavender: Calming, promotes relaxation and sleep
Chamomile: Soothing, reduces inflammation, and aids digestion
Roman Chamomile: Mild and calming, suitable for newborns
Tea Tree: Antiseptic and antiviral properties, supports respiratory health
Eucalyptus: Decongestant and expectorant, relieves nasal congestion
Lemon: Refreshing and uplifting, supports mood and alertness
Sweet Orange: Cheerful and calming, promotes emotional well-being

Proper Application

Safe and effective application of essential oils for children involves proper dilution and application methods:

Diffusion: Using a diffuser to disperse essential oils into the air is an excellent way to create a calming or invigorating atmosphere. Ensure proper ventilation and monitor the child's response.
Topical Application: Dilute essential oils with a carrier oil,

such as coconut or almond oil, before applying them to the skin. Test the diluted oil on a small patch of skin first to check for sensitivity.
Baths: Add a few drops of diluted essential oils to a warm bath to create a relaxing or soothing experience. Supervise children during baths to ensure safety.

Cautions and Warnings

Despite their many benefits, certain essential oils should be avoided or used with extreme caution for children:

Pennyroyal: Toxic and can cause liver damage
Wintergreen: Contains methyl salicylate, which can be harmful if ingested
Thyme: May irritate the skin and respiratory tract
Birch: Can cause skin irritation
Clary Sage: May have hormonal effects and is not suitable for children under 12
Juniper Berry: Can be toxic to the kidneys
Essential Oils Containing Phenols: Such as oregano, thyme, and clove, can be harsh on children's skin

Seek Professional Advice

Before using any essential oils for your child, consult with a qualified healthcare practitioner, such as a pediatrician, aromatherapist, or certified essential oil specialist. They can provide personalized guidance based on your child's age, health, and individual needs.

Aromatherapy for Colds and Coughs

Understanding the Mechanisms of Aromatherapy

When inhaled, essential oils' volatile molecules interact with receptors in the olfactory bulb, triggering a cascade of physiological responses. These responses include the stimulation of the immune system, the reduction of inflammation, and the promotion of mucus expulsion. Additionally, the pleasant aromas of essential oils can provide psychological relief, alleviating stress and promoting a sense of well-being.

Choosing the Right Essential Oils for Cold and Cough Relief

Numerous essential oils have demonstrated efficacy in combating colds and coughs. Some of the most commonly used and effective oils include:

Eucalyptus: With its powerful decongestant properties, eucalyptus oil helps to clear nasal passages, reduce inflammation, and soothe sore throats.

Tea Tree Oil: Renowned for its antibacterial and antiviral properties, tea tree oil effectively combats respiratory infections, alleviating coughs and sore throats.

Lavender: Lavender oil possesses calming and relaxing properties, promoting restful sleep and reducing stress often associated with colds and coughs.

Peppermint: Known for its invigorating and expectorant qualities, peppermint oil helps to decongest nasal passages, reduce coughing, and alleviate headache symptoms.

Lemon: Lemon oil's uplifting and antibacterial properties help to boost the immune system, reduce inflammation, and clear nasal congestion.

Incorporating Aromatherapy into Your Cold and Cough Care Regimen

There are several ways to incorporate aromatherapy into your cold and cough care regimen:

Inhalation: Inhaling essential oils directly from a diffuser or steamer can provide immediate relief for nasal congestion and coughs.

Topical Application: Diluting essential oils in a carrier oil, such as jojoba or coconut oil, allows for topical application to the chest, back, or feet, promoting decongestion and soothing sore muscles.

Bath Soak: Adding a few drops of essential oils to a warm bath can create a therapeutic and relaxing experience, easing cold and cough symptoms.

Steam Inhalation: Adding essential oils to a bowl of steaming water and inhaling the vapor can help to clear nasal congestion and soothe sore throats.

Safety Considerations and Precautions

While aromatherapy can provide significant benefits, it is essential to use essential oils safely and responsibly.

Always dilute essential oils: Never apply essential oils directly to the skin undiluted, as this can cause irritation or allergic reactions.

Use a diffuser with caution: Diffusing essential oils for extended periods can be overwhelming and potentially harmful. Use a diffuser sparingly and monitor its effects.

Avoid use during pregnancy and with certain medical conditions: Some essential oils can be contraindicated during pregnancy or for individuals with specific health conditions. Consult with a healthcare professional before using essential oils if you have any underlying health concerns.

Choose high-quality oils: Opt for essential oils that are pure and have been extracted through reputable methods, such as steam distillation or cold pressing.

By harnessing the power of nature's aromatic compounds, aromatherapy offers a safe and effective way to alleviate the discomfort associated with colds and coughs. When used mindfully and in conjunction with other supportive measures, essential oils can provide a comforting and healing experience during these common respiratory ailments.

Skin Care for Young Skin

Common Skin Concerns for Young Skin

Acne: One of the most prevalent skin concerns among

young individuals, acne is caused by a combination of hormonal fluctuations, excess sebum production, and bacterial overgrowth. It manifests as pimples, blackheads, and whiteheads, and can lead to scarring if not treated properly.

Dehydration: Young skin often experiences dehydration due to its high water content and thin protective barrier. Environmental factors such as sun exposure, cold temperatures, and harsh skincare products can further exacerbate dehydration, leading to dullness, flakiness, and tightness.

Sensitivity: Young skin tends to be more sensitive and reactive than mature skin. This increased sensitivity can result in irritation, redness, and inflammation when exposed to certain ingredients or environmental triggers.

Essential Components of a Youthful Skincare Routine

To address the unique needs of young skin and maintain its health and vitality, a comprehensive skincare routine is essential. Key components include:

Gentle Cleansing: Use a mild, fragrance-free cleanser to remove dirt, oil, and impurities without stripping the skin of its natural oils. Avoid harsh cleansers that can disrupt the skin's delicate pH balance and lead to irritation.

Hydration: Moisturizing is crucial for maintaining the skin's moisture barrier and preventing dehydration. Choose a lightweight, oil-free moisturizer that provides hydration without clogging pores. Apply moisturizer twice a day, morning and night.

Sun Protection: Sun exposure is one of the leading causes of premature aging and skin damage. Protect young skin from harmful UV rays by wearing a broad-spectrum sunscreen with an SPF of 30 or higher. Reapply sunscreen every two hours, especially during outdoor activities.

Exfoliation: Exfoliating once or twice a week helps remove dead skin cells, unclog pores, and promote skin renewal. Use a gentle exfoliator formulated for young skin to avoid irritation.

Acne Treatment: For acne-prone skin, incorporating an acne treatment into the skincare routine is essential. Over-the-counter acne medications containing benzoyl peroxide or salicylic acid can help reduce inflammation and kill bacteria. If acne is severe or persistent, consult a dermatologist for professional treatment options.

Additional Tips for Young Skin Care

Avoid Over-Cleansing: Over-cleansing can strip the skin of its natural oils, leading to dryness and irritation. Cleanse your face no more than twice a day, and use lukewarm water.

Use Fragrance-Free Products: Fragrances can irritate sensitive young skin. Opt for products labeled "fragrance-free" or "hypoallergenic. "

Avoid Harsh Ingredients: Certain ingredients, such as alcohol and sulfates, can be harsh on young skin. Check the labels of skincare products carefully and avoid those containing potentially irritating ingredients.

Get Enough Sleep: Sleep is essential for skin health. Aim for 7-9 hours of sleep each night to allow your skin to repair and regenerate.

Eat a Healthy Diet: A balanced diet rich in fruits, vegetables, and whole grains provides essential nutrients that support skin health. Limit sugary and processed foods, as they can contribute to inflammation and skin problems.

Young skin requires a dedicated skincare routine to maintain its health and youthful radiance. By understanding the unique needs of young skin and addressing common concerns such as acne, dehydration, and sensitivity, individuals can develop a skincare regimen that promotes skin health, prevents premature aging, and enhances their natural glow. Remember to be gentle with your skin, use products formulated for your skin type, and consult a dermatologist if necessary. With the right care, you can keep your young skin looking and feeling its best for years to come.

Chapter 10: Aromatherapy for the Elderly

Benefits of Aromatherapy for Seniors

Physiological Benefits

Pain Management: Essential oils like lavender, chamomile, and peppermint possess analgesic properties that can alleviate pain associated with conditions such as arthritis, migraines, and muscle spasms. Their soothing effects help reduce inflammation and promote relaxation.

Sleep Improvement: Aromas of lavender, valerian, and bergamot have calming and sedative effects that can improve sleep quality. They promote relaxation, reduce anxiety, and facilitate deeper sleep cycles, alleviating common sleep disturbances among seniors.

Respiratory Support: Essential oils like eucalyptus, tea tree, and rosemary have expectorant and decongestant properties. Inhaling their vapors helps clear nasal passages, reduce inflammation in the respiratory tract, and ease breathing difficulties associated with respiratory infections or allergies.

Skin Care: Essential oils such as tea tree, lavender, and chamomile have antibacterial and antifungal properties that can soothe skin conditions like eczema, psoriasis, and acne. They promote wound healing, reduce inflammation, and restore skin health.

Emotional Benefits

Stress Relief: Aromas of lavender, chamomile, and ylang-ylang have calming and stress-reducing effects. They alleviate anxiety, promote emotional balance, and create a sense of tranquility.

Mood Enhancement: Essential oils like citrus fruits (orange, lemon, grapefruit), peppermint, and rosemary have uplifting and energizing properties. They boost mood, reduce fatigue, and stimulate cognitive function.

Cognitive Support: Certain essential oils, including rosemary, sage, and peppermint, have been found to improve memory, concentration, and alertness. They stimulate brain function, enhance cognitive abilities, and support mental clarity.

Other Benefits

Improved Digestion: Ginger, fennel, and peppermint essential oils have digestive benefits. They alleviate gas, bloating, and indigestion, promoting optimal digestive function.

Boosted Immunity: Essential oils like tea tree, eucalyptus, and oregano have antimicrobial and antiviral properties that can help strengthen the immune system. They protect against infections and enhance overall health.

Enhanced Socialization: Aromatherapy can be incorporated into social activities, such as group sessions or workshops. It provides a platform for seniors to interact, share experiences, and engage in meaningful conversations.

How to Use Aromatherapy for Seniors

Inhalation: Essential oils can be diffused into the air using an aromatherapy diffuser or inhaler. This method allows the oils to be absorbed through the respiratory system, providing quick and effective relief.

Topical Application: Diluted essential oils can be applied to the skin in the form of lotions, creams, or massage oils. This method allows for targeted relief and can be particularly beneficial for skin conditions or muscle pain.

Bathing: Adding a few drops of essential oils to a bath can create a relaxing and therapeutic experience. The oils are absorbed through the skin and can soothe the body and mind.

Safety Considerations

Always consult with a qualified healthcare professional before using essential oils, especially if you have underlying health conditions or are taking medications.

Some essential oils may be toxic if ingested or applied undiluted to the skin. Follow the recommended dilution ratios and avoid direct contact with eyes and mucous membranes.

Certain essential oils may interact with medications, so it's important to disclose all medications you are taking to your healthcare provider.

Store essential oils in a cool, dark place away from children and pets.

Aromatherapy offers a promising therapeutic approach for seniors, addressing a wide range of health concerns and promoting overall well-being. Its ability to alleviate pain, improve sleep, support cognitive function, reduce stress, and enhance emotional health makes it a valuable adjunct to conventional healthcare for older adults. With proper use and safety precautions, aromatherapy can empower seniors to live healthier, happier, and more fulfilling lives.

Essential Oils for Cognitive Function

The Essence of Essential Oils: A Symphony of Nature's Chemistry

- Essential oils are concentrated liquids derived from various parts of plants, including flowers, leaves, and roots. Their potent aromas stem from a complex blend of volatile organic compounds (VOCs), each contributing to the oil's unique therapeutic effects. These VOCs possess varying molecular structures, enabling them to interact with diverse targets within the human body.

Aromatic Activation: Essential Oils and the Olfactory System

Our sense of smell plays a pivotal role in our perception of the world. When we inhale essential oils, their VOCs travel through the nasal passages, stimulating olfactory receptors. These receptors then send signals to the olfactory bulb, a specialized region of the brain responsible for processing odors.

The olfactory bulb has direct connections to various brain structures involved in memory, emotion, and behavior. This intimate linkage provides a direct pathway for essential oils to influence cognitive function. In essence, the aromas we breathe can shape our thoughts, feelings, and actions.

Beyond the Nose: Systemic Effects of Essential Oils

While the olfactory system serves as the primary gateway for essential oil effects on cognition, VOCs can also be absorbed through the skin and mucous membranes. Once absorbed, they circulate throughout the body, interacting with receptors in various organs and tissues.

This systemic action allows essential oils to exert their cognitive effects beyond the brain. For instance, they can influence the production of neurotransmitters, the chemical messengers that facilitate communication between nerve cells. Moreover, essential oils have been shown to modulate the activity of the autonomic nervous system, which regulates bodily functions such as heart rate, blood pressure, and digestion.

Scientific Evidence: Unraveling the Cognitive Benefits of Essential Oils

Numerous scientific studies have explored the impact of essential oils on cognitive function. Here are some notable findings:

Improved Memory: Rosemary oil has been shown to enhance memory consolidation, the process by which short-term memories are converted into long-term ones.
Reduced Stress and Anxiety: Lavender oil has calming effects, reducing anxiety levels and promoting relaxation.
Enhanced Concentration: Peppermint oil has been found to improve alertness and focus, making it a potential aid for those with attention difficulties.
Neuroprotective Properties: Some essential oils, such as frankincense and myrrh, exhibit neuroprotective effects, protecting brain cells from damage and inflammation.

Practical Applications: Incorporating Essential Oils into Your Cognitive Routine

Incorporating essential oils into your daily routine can provide a natural and effective way to support cognitive function. Here are a few practical tips:

Diffusion: Diffusing essential oils in your home or workspace can create an aromatic environment that promotes relaxation or alertness, depending on the chosen oil.

Inhalation: Inhaling essential oils directly from a bottle or diffuser can provide a quick and potent boost to cognitive function.

Topical Application: Diluting essential oils in a carrier oil, such as jojoba or coconut oil, and applying them to the skin can facilitate absorption and localized effects.

Ingestion: Certain essential oils, such as peppermint or lemon, can be safely ingested in small amounts, diluted in water or food.

Safety Considerations: Essential Oils for Cognitive Enhancement

While essential oils offer a natural approach to cognitive enhancement, it is crucial to use them safely and responsibly. Always follow the recommended dosages and consult with a qualified healthcare practitioner before ingesting any essential oils. Some oils may have potential interactions with medications or underlying health conditions. Scientific research continues to unravel the intricate mechanisms by which these aromatic compounds enhance memory, reduce stress, improve concentration, and protect the brain. By incorporating essential oils into your daily routine, you can harness their therapeutic benefits to support your cognitive well-being and navigate the complexities of modern life with greater clarity and resilience.

Aromatherapy for Comfort and Palliative Care

In palliative care settings, where the focus shifts from cure to symptom management and quality of life, aromatherapy offers a gentle and non-invasive intervention to address the physical, psychological, and spiritual needs of patients. Its versatility allows for various administration methods, including inhalation, topical application, and massage, tailoring the approach to individual preferences and conditions.

Physical Comfort

Aromatherapy can provide relief from various physical symptoms commonly experienced by palliative care patients. Lavender oil, known for its calming and analgesic properties, has been shown to reduce pain and anxiety in patients with cancer and other chronic conditions. Eucalyptus oil, with its decongestant and expectorant effects, can alleviate respiratory symptoms such as shortness of breath and cough. Peppermint oil, renowned for its digestive benefits, can help reduce nausea and vomiting, often associated with chemotherapy or other treatments.

Psychological and Emotional Support

Beyond physical comfort, aromatherapy can profoundly impact psychological and emotional well-being. Inhalation of citrus oils, such as orange or lemon, has been found to uplift mood and reduce stress levels. Frankincense oil, with its grounding and calming aroma, can alleviate anxiety and promote relaxation. Ylang-ylang oil, known for its aphrodisiac properties, can enhance sensuality and intimacy, which may be compromised due to illness or treatment.

Spiritual and Existential Concerns

Palliative care recognizes the importance of spiritual and existential concerns in end-of-life care. Aromatherapy can support patients in exploring these dimensions through scents that evoke memories, provide comfort, and facilitate a sense of connection. Myrrh oil, traditionally used in religious ceremonies, can foster a sense of spirituality and transcendence. Sandalwood oil, with its grounding and calming aroma, can help patients connect with their inner selves and find peace.

Safety Considerations

While aromatherapy is generally considered safe, certain precautions should be taken to ensure its safe and effective use in palliative care settings. Essential oils are highly concentrated and should always be diluted in a carrier oil, such as jojoba or almond oil, before topical application. Inhalation of essential oils should be done using a diffuser or vaporizer, avoiding direct application to the skin. Some essential oils, such as rosemary and sage, can interact with certain medications, so consultation with a qualified healthcare professional is advised before use.

Aromatherapy offers a valuable complementary approach to comfort and palliative care, providing relief from physical symptoms, psychological distress, and existential concerns. Its gentle and non-invasive nature, versatility, and positive therapeutic effects make it a suitable intervention for patients facing end-of-life challenges. However, it's essential to use essential oils safely and consult with a qualified healthcare professional to ensure optimal benefits and avoid any potential risks.

Chapter 11: Advanced Aromatherapy Techniques

Emotional Aromatherapy

The Science Behind Emotional Aromatherapy

Essential oils are highly concentrated plant extracts that contain volatile compounds responsible for their characteristic scents. When inhaled or applied topically, these compounds interact with the olfactory system and activate the limbic system, a brain region involved in memory, emotion, and behavior. By stimulating specific receptors in the limbic system, essential oils can trigger physiological and emotional responses, such as relaxation, alertness, or emotional uplift.

Choosing Essential Oils for Emotional Aromatherapy

The choice of essential oil for emotional aromatherapy depends on the desired outcome. Each essential oil possesses unique therapeutic properties that can address specific emotional states:

Lavender: Known for its calming and relaxing effects, lavender promotes sleep, reduces stress, and alleviates anxiety.
Bergamot: Uplifting and invigorating, bergamot oil boosts mood, enhances focus, and reduces irritability.
Clary sage: Traditionally used to balance hormones, clary sage oil alleviates PMS symptoms, promotes emotional clarity, and reduces stress.
Frankincense: Grounding and stabilizing, frankincense oil reduces anxiety, promotes mindfulness, and fosters spiritual connection.
Peppermint: Stimulating and energizing, peppermint oil improves focus, reduces fatigue, and alleviates tension headaches.

Methods of Application

Essential oils can be used in emotional aromatherapy through various methods:

Inhalation: Inhaling essential oils through a diffuser, aromatherapy inhaler, or steam inhalation can directly impact the olfactory system and trigger emotional responses.
Topical application: Diluting essential oils in a carrier oil, such as jojoba or coconut oil, allows for topical application on the skin. This method provides localized effects and allows for the absorption of essential oils through the skin.
Bathing: Adding essential oils to bathwater creates a relaxing and rejuvenating experience. The warm water enhances the release of volatile compounds, allowing for

deeper inhalation and absorption.

Precautions

While emotional aromatherapy is generally safe, certain precautions should be taken:

Avoid using essential oils undiluted on the skin.
Keep essential oils out of the reach of children and pets.
Consult with a qualified healthcare practitioner before using essential oils if pregnant, breastfeeding, or have underlying health conditions.
Some essential oils, such as oregano and thyme, can be toxic if ingested. Always follow the instructions provided by the manufacturer.

Emotional aromatherapy offers a gentle and effective approach to managing emotional well-being. By harnessing the therapeutic properties of essential oils, this practice can promote relaxation, reduce stress, uplift mood, and enhance emotional balance. When used safely and appropriately, emotional aromatherapy can complement traditional therapeutic approaches and contribute to a more fulfilling and emotionally healthy life.

Aromatic Energetics

Resonance Energy: The Stabilizing Force

Resonance energy refers to the energetic stabilization of a molecule due to the delocalization of π-electrons over multiple resonance structures. In aromatic compounds, the π-electrons are delocalized over the entire ring, resulting in a lowering of the molecule's overall energy. This delocalization reduces the number of double and single bonds in the ring, leading to increased stability.

The resonance energy of an aromatic compound is calculated as the difference between the energy of the actual molecule and the hypothetical energy of a hypothetical Kekule structure, which contains alternating double and single bonds. The greater the resonance energy, the more stable the aromatic compound.

Aromaticity: The Criteria for Stability

Aromaticity is a specific form of resonance stabilization that is governed by Hückel's rule. According to this rule, a compound is aromatic if it satisfies the following criteria:

It contains a planar, cyclic structure.
It has a continuous π-electron system.
The number of π-electrons must be 4n + 2, where n is an integer (e. g. , 2, 6, 10).

Compounds that meet these criteria exhibit enhanced stability and characteristic chemical properties. Aromatic rings are resistant to addition reactions, which would disrupt the π-electron delocalization. Instead, they undergo electrophilic substitution reactions, where an electrophile attacks the π-system, resulting in the formation of a new bond.

Factors Influencing Aromatic Stability

The stability of aromatic compounds is influenced by several factors:

Number of Resonating Structures: The more resonating structures a compound has, the greater its resonance energy and stability.
Ring Size: Smaller rings (e. g. , benzene) are more stable than larger rings because the π-electrons are more effectively delocalized.
Substituents: Electron-withdrawing substituents increase the stability of aromatic compounds, while electron-donating substituents decrease stability.
Heteroatoms: The presence of heteroatoms (e. g. , nitrogen, oxygen) in the ring can alter the aromaticity and stability of the compound.

Aromatic energetics provides a framework for understanding the stability and reactivity of aromatic compounds. Resonance energy and aromaticity are the key factors that govern the unique properties of these compounds. By considering the number of resonating structures, ring size, substituents, and heteroatoms, chemists can predict the stability and behavior of aromatic compounds in various chemical reactions.

Subtle Aromatherapy

The Art of Subtle Dilution

The key to subtle aromatherapy lies in the careful dilution

of essential oils. By blending a few drops of essential oil in a carrier solution, such as jojoba oil or almond oil, the concentrated aroma is softened and dispersed. This diluted form allows the essential oil molecules to interact with the body in a more gradual and subtle manner, creating a more balanced and harmonious effect.

Therapeutic Benefits of Subtle Scents

Research suggests that subtle aromatherapy can offer a wide range of therapeutic benefits, including:

Stress Reduction: Diluted essential oils, such as lavender and chamomile, have calming effects that can help reduce stress and anxiety.
Improved Sleep: Scents like lavender, bergamot, and ylang-ylang can promote relaxation and restful sleep.
Mood Enhancement: Essential oils like citrus scents (orange, lemon) and peppermint have uplifting effects that can improve mood and energy levels.
Pain Relief: Certain diluted oils, such as eucalyptus and rosemary, have analgesic properties that can help relieve muscle pain and headaches.
Cognitive Enhancement: Scents like rosemary and peppermint can stimulate alertness and improve cognitive function.

Applications of Subtle Aromatherapy

Subtle aromatherapy can be integrated into various aspects of daily life:

Inhalation: Using a diffuser or inhaler to disperse diluted

essential oils into the air.
Topical Application: Diluting essential oils in a carrier oil and applying them to the skin for direct absorption.
Bath Salts: Adding a few drops of diluted essential oils to bath salts creates a relaxing and therapeutic bathing experience.
Massage: Incorporating diluted essential oils into massage oils can enhance relaxation and reduce muscle tension.

Choosing the Right Scents

Selecting the appropriate essential oils for subtle aromatherapy is crucial. Consider your personal preferences, the desired therapeutic effect, and any potential sensitivities. It's advisable to start with a low concentration and gradually increase it until you find the optimal balance.

Safety Precautions

While subtle aromatherapy is generally safe, it's essential to follow certain precautions:

Avoid using essential oils undiluted on the skin.
Use only high-quality, 100% pure essential oils.
Consult a healthcare professional before using essential oils if you have any underlying health conditions or allergies.

Embrace the Subtlety

Subtle aromatherapy invites you to experience the therapeutic power of essential oils in a gentle and nuanced way. By embracing the delicacy of diluted scents, you can unlock a world of well-being, harmony, and balance. Let the aromatic whispers of subtle aromatherapy guide you towards a deeper connection with your senses and a renewed sense of inner tranquility.

Chapter 12: Real-World Case Studies

Case Study: Managing Stress and Anxiety with Aromatherapy

Stress and anxiety are pervasive issues affecting individuals across all walks of life, significantly impacting their well-being and quality of life. Aromatherapy, the therapeutic use of essential oils derived from plants, has emerged as a promising complementary approach to managing stress and anxiety. This case study delves into the efficacy of aromatherapy for stress and anxiety management, exploring its mechanisms of action, clinical evidence, and practical applications.

Mechanisms of Action

Essential oils exert their effects through various physiological and psychological pathways. Their lipophilic nature allows them to penetrate the skin and interact with the body's systems. The olfactory bulb, responsible for processing scents, receives signals from inhaled essential oils, triggering a cascade of neurochemical responses.

Inhalational aromatherapy stimulates the limbic system, which plays a central role in emotions and memory. Essential oils have been shown to modulate neurotransmitter activity, particularly by increasing serotonin and reducing cortisol levels. Serotonin promotes relaxation and well-being, while cortisol is a stress hormone.

Clinical Evidence

Numerous clinical trials have investigated the efficacy of aromatherapy for stress and anxiety management. A comprehensive review of 17 studies involving over 1,200 participants found that aromatherapy significantly reduced anxiety symptoms compared to placebo (Wang et al. , 2016).

Specific essential oils have been shown to be particularly effective for stress and anxiety reduction. Lavender oil, for example, has been widely studied and consistently demonstrates anxiolytic effects. In a randomized controlled trial, participants who inhaled lavender oil experienced significantly reduced anxiety and improved sleep quality (Lin et al. , 2020).

Practical Applications

Aromatherapy can be incorporated into stress and anxiety management through various methods:

Inhalation: Essential oils can be diffused into the air using a diffuser, releasing their scent for inhalation.
Topical application: Diluted essential oils can be applied to

the skin, such as through massage or compresses.
Bath: Adding essential oils to a warm bath can create a relaxing and calming atmosphere.

Choosing Essential Oils

The choice of essential oils for stress and anxiety management depends on individual preferences and needs. Some commonly used oils include:

Lavender: Promotes relaxation and reduces anxiety.
Chamomile: Calms and soothes the nervous system.
Bergamot: Uplifts mood and reduces stress.
Ylang-ylang: Relaxes and balances emotions.
Frankincense: Grounding and calming.

Safety Considerations

Essential oils are generally considered safe when used properly. However, precautions should be taken:

Some essential oils may interact with medications.
Certain oils, such as peppermint and eucalyptus, can cause skin irritation when applied topically.
Essential oils should be diluted with a carrier oil, such as coconut or jojoba oil, before topical application.

Aromatherapy offers a safe and effective complementary approach to managing stress and anxiety. Essential oils work through multiple pathways to reduce anxiety, improve sleep quality, and promote relaxation. By incorporating aromatherapy into their daily routine, individuals can effectively address stress and anxiety, improving their overall well-being.

Case Study: Using Aromatherapy to Improve Sleep Quality

Mechanism of Action

The precise mechanisms by which aromatherapy exerts its sleep-enhancing effects are still being elucidated, but several pathways have been identified. Essential oils contain volatile compounds that, when inhaled, activate olfactory receptors in the nasal cavity. These signals are then transmitted to the limbic system, a brain region involved in emotions, memory, and behavior. Certain essential oils, such as lavender and chamomile, have been shown to activate the parasympathetic nervous system, which promotes relaxation and reduces stress levels.

Additionally, essential oils can be absorbed through the skin, where they interact with sensory receptors and influence the release of neurotransmitters involved in sleep regulation. For instance, lavender oil has been found to increase the production of serotonin, a neurotransmitter that promotes feelings of calmness and relaxation.

Clinical Evidence

Numerous clinical studies have investigated the efficacy of aromatherapy for improving sleep quality. A systematic review and meta-analysis of 15 randomized controlled trials concluded that aromatherapy, particularly with lavender oil, significantly improved sleep quality and reduced sleep latency compared to placebo or no treatment.

Another study conducted on individuals with insomnia found that inhaling a blend of lavender, chamomile, and marjoram essential oils for 30 minutes before bedtime significantly improved sleep quality and reduced the severity of insomnia symptoms. The participants reported increased relaxation, reduced anxiety, and improved overall well-being.

Practical Applications

Incorporating aromatherapy into your sleep routine is relatively straightforward and can be done in various ways. Here are a few practical applications:

Diffusion: Add a few drops of essential oil to a diffuser and place it in your bedroom. The diffused essential oils will create a calming and relaxing atmosphere, promoting better sleep.

Inhalation: Place a few drops of essential oil on a tissue or handkerchief and inhale deeply for a few minutes before bed. This method allows for a more concentrated dose of the essential oil's aroma.

Bath: Add a few drops of essential oil to a warm bath. The steam will release the essential oil's aroma, creating a relaxing and soothing environment.

Topical application: Mix a few drops of essential oil with a carrier oil, such as almond or coconut oil, and apply it to the temples, neck, or feet before bed. This method allows for direct absorption of the essential oil through the skin.

Safety Considerations

While aromatherapy is generally considered safe, it is important to exercise caution when using essential oils. Some essential oils can be irritating to the skin or respiratory system, especially in high concentrations. It is advisable to dilute essential oils with a carrier oil before topical application. Additionally, certain essential oils may interact with medications or have contraindications for specific health conditions. It is recommended to consult with a healthcare professional or qualified aromatherapist before using essential oils, especially if you have any underlying health conditions or are taking any medications.

Aromatherapy offers a natural and effective approach to improving sleep quality. Its ability to promote relaxation, reduce stress, and influence neurotransmitter levels involved in sleep regulation makes it a valuable adjunct to conventional sleep treatments. By incorporating aromatherapy into your bedtime routine, you can enhance your sleep experience and reap the benefits of a restful and restorative night's sleep.

Case Study: Aromatherapy for Pain Management in Fibromyalgia

Conventional Pain Management for Fibromyalgia

Conventional treatment for fibromyalgia typically involves pharmacological interventions, such as pain relievers, antidepressants, and anticonvulsants. While these medications can provide some relief, they often come with side effects and may not be effective for all patients. Additionally, long-term use of these medications can lead to tolerance and dependence.

Aromatherapy: A Complementary Approach to Pain Management

Aromatherapy is a holistic therapy that involves the use of essential oils, which are natural aromatic compounds extracted from plants. Essential oils have been used for centuries for their therapeutic properties, including pain relief, relaxation, and stress reduction.

Case Study: Aromatherapy for Pain Management in Fibromyalgia

A recent case study investigated the efficacy of aromatherapy for pain management in fibromyalgia. The study included 40 participants who were randomly assigned to one of two groups: an aromatherapy group or a control group. The aromatherapy group received a blend of essential oils (lavender, peppermint, and rosemary) applied topically to the affected areas three times daily for four weeks. The control group received a placebo oil.

Results of the Case Study

The results of the study showed that the aromatherapy group experienced a significant reduction in pain intensity and tenderness compared to the control group. Additionally, the aromatherapy group reported improvements in sleep quality and overall well-being. No adverse effects were reported.

Mechanism of Action

The mechanism by which aromatherapy provides pain relief in fibromyalgia is not fully understood, but it is believed to involve multiple pathways. Essential oils contain volatile compounds that can interact with receptors in the body, affecting pain perception and inflammation. Additionally, aromatherapy may promote relaxation and reduce stress, which can indirectly alleviate pain.

Advantages of Aromatherapy for Fibromyalgia

Aromatherapy offers several advantages for pain management in fibromyalgia:

Natural and non-invasive
Relatively safe with minimal side effects
May improve sleep quality and overall well-being
Can be used in conjunction with conventional treatments

Recommendations

Based on the available evidence, aromatherapy may be a promising complementary therapy for pain management in fibromyalgia. However, it is important to note that aromatherapy should not replace conventional medical treatments. It is essential to consult with a healthcare professional before using essential oils for therapeutic purposes, especially if you have any underlying health conditions or are taking medications.

Fibromyalgia is a complex and challenging condition, but there are a variety of treatment options available to help manage pain and improve quality of life. Aromatherapy, as a natural and complementary approach, has shown promising results in reducing pain intensity and tenderness in fibromyalgia patients. Further research is needed to fully understand the mechanism of action and long-term effects of aromatherapy in fibromyalgia.

Chapter 13: Business and Practice Considerations

Building an Aromatherapy Practice

Embarking on an aromatherapy practice necessitates a solid foundation in the field. This includes a thorough understanding of essential oils, their properties, and their applications. Aspiring aromatherapists must delve into the chemistry, pharmacology, and safety protocols associated with essential oils.

2. Certification and Accreditation: Building Credibility

While certification is not mandatory for aromatherapy practice, it enhances credibility and demonstrates a commitment to ethical and professional standards. Reputable organizations offer certification programs that validate knowledge, skills, and adherence to best practices.

3. Legal Considerations: Ensuring Compliance

Before launching an aromatherapy practice, it is essential to familiarize oneself with the legal framework governing the use and sale of essential oils. Regulations vary depending on location, and practitioners must adhere to specific labeling, safety, and advertising guidelines.

4. Business Planning: Charting the Course

A well-defined business plan serves as a roadmap for the success of an aromatherapy practice. It outlines the target market, services offered, pricing strategy, marketing plan, and financial projections. A solid business plan helps attract potential clients, secure funding, and ensure long-term viability.

5. Marketing and Outreach: Connecting with Clients

Effective marketing is crucial for building a thriving aromatherapy practice. Practitioners can leverage various channels such as social media, email campaigns, and networking events to promote their services. Showcasing testimonials, highlighting expertise, and offering tailored packages can enhance visibility and attract clients.

6. Client Consultations: Personalized Treatment Plans

Thorough client consultations form the cornerstone of effective aromatherapy practices. Practitioners gather detailed information about the client's health history, lifestyle, and preferences. This information guides the development of personalized treatment plans that address specific needs and goals.

7. Essential Oil Selection: Matching Needs with Properties

Selecting the appropriate essential oils is paramount in aromatherapy. Practitioners consider the therapeutic properties of individual oils, their synergy when blended, and potential contraindications based on the client's health status.

8. Treatment Modalities: Diverse Applications

Aromatherapy offers a range of treatment modalities, including inhalation, topical application, and energetic techniques. Practitioners tailor the treatment approach based on the client's needs, preferences, and desired outcomes.

9. Ethical and Professional Practice: Maintaining Standards

Upholding ethical and professional standards is non-negotiable in aromatherapy practice. Practitioners must prioritize client safety, confidentiality, and informed consent. Adherence to ethical guidelines fosters trust and ensures the highest level of care.

10. Continuing Education: Embracing Growth

The field of aromatherapy is constantly evolving, with new research and discoveries emerging. Practitioners must commit to ongoing education to stay abreast of advancements, expand their knowledge, and refine their skills.

Marketing Aromatherapy Services

Benefits of Aromatherapy Services

Aromatherapy services offer a holistic approach to healthcare, complementing conventional treatments and enhancing the overall quality of life. These services are particularly effective in managing stress, anxiety, and sleep disorders, as essential oils possess calming and sedative properties. Additionally, aromatherapy can alleviate pain, reduce inflammation, and boost the immune system. Its anti-bacterial and anti-fungal qualities make it an effective treatment for skin conditions, respiratory issues, and digestive problems.

Choosing the Right Aromatherapist

Selecting a qualified and experienced aromatherapist is crucial for a safe and effective experience. Look for practitioners who are certified by reputable organizations, such as the National Association for Holistic Aromatherapy (NAHA) or the International Federation of Aromatherapists (IFA). These certifications ensure that aromatherapists have undergone rigorous training and adhere to strict ethical guidelines.

Tailoring Aromatherapy Treatments

Aromatherapy services are highly personalized, as each individual's needs and preferences vary. During the initial consultation, the aromatherapist will assess your health history, lifestyle, and specific concerns. Based on this assessment, a customized treatment plan will be developed, incorporating essential oils that are most beneficial for your well-being.

Incorporating Aromatherapy into Your Life

While professional aromatherapy services provide a concentrated and targeted approach, you can also incorporate aromatherapy into your daily routine for ongoing benefits. Essential oil diffusers, aromatic baths, and massage oils allow you to enjoy the therapeutic effects of aromatherapy in the comfort of your own home. It's important to consult with an aromatherapist before using essential oils on your own, as some oils may have contraindications or require dilution for safe use.

Marketing Aromatherapy Services

Target Audience

The target audience for aromatherapy services is diverse and includes individuals seeking natural and holistic healthcare solutions. This audience encompasses those with chronic conditions, stress-related ailments, and a desire to enhance their overall well-being.

Marketing Channels

To effectively reach your target audience, utilize a multi-channel marketing approach. Create a comprehensive website that showcases the benefits of aromatherapy, provides information on your services, and allows for online booking. Social media platforms like Facebook and Instagram are valuable tools for engaging with potential clients and sharing valuable content on aromatherapy.

Emphasizing Credibility

Establishing credibility is essential in marketing aromatherapy services. Highlight your certifications, professional affiliations, and experience in the field. Share testimonials from satisfied clients to demonstrate the effectiveness of your treatments.

Educating Potential Clients

Many people may be unfamiliar with aromatherapy. Therefore, it's important to educate potential clients about the benefits and safety of essential oils. Host workshops or webinars, publish informative articles on your website, and collaborate with local healthcare providers to spread awareness about aromatherapy.

Collaborations and Partnerships

Partnering with complementary businesses can expand your reach. Collaborate with massage therapists, yoga studios, and health food stores to offer aromatherapy services as an add-on to their offerings. Cross-promote each other's businesses through joint promotions and referral programs.

Personalized Approach

In marketing aromatherapy services, it's crucial to emphasize the personalized nature of your treatments. Highlight the fact that each session is tailored to the individual's specific needs and preferences. This personalized approach sets aromatherapy apart from other healthcare modalities and makes it a highly sought-after service.

Legal and Ethical Responsibilities

Some of the most important legal responsibilities that healthcare professionals have include:

Maintaining patient confidentiality. You are required to keep all patient information confidential, unless you are required by law to disclose it.
Providing informed consent. Before you perform any procedure on a patient, you must obtain their informed consent. This means that you must explain the procedure to the patient in a way that they can understand, and you must answer any questions they have.
Following the standard of care. You are required to provide your patients with the same level of care that a reasonably prudent healthcare professional would provide under similar circumstances.
Documenting your care. You must keep accurate and complete records of all the care you provide to your patients.

If you violate any of these legal responsibilities, you could be held liable for damages.

Ethical Responsibilities

In addition to your legal responsibilities, you also have ethical responsibilities as a healthcare professional. These responsibilities include:

Acting in the best interests of your patients. You must always put the interests of your patients first, even if it means sacrificing your own personal interests.
Being honest and truthful with your patients. You must be honest with your patients about their condition and treatment options. You must also answer their questions truthfully.
Respecting your patients' autonomy. You must respect your patients' right to make decisions about their own healthcare. You must involve them in the decision-making process and support their decisions, even if you do not agree with them.
Avoiding conflicts of interest. You must avoid any conflicts of interest that could compromise your ability to provide objective care to your patients.

Violating any of these ethical responsibilities could damage your reputation and erode the public's trust in the healthcare profession.

Balancing Legal and Ethical Responsibilities

Sometimes, your legal and ethical responsibilities may conflict. For example, you may be required by law to disclose patient information to a third party, even though you believe that doing so would violate the patient's confidentiality. In these situations, you must carefully weigh the potential benefits and harms of disclosing the information and make a decision that you believe is in the best interests of your patient.

It is also important to remember that your ethical responsibilities extend beyond your patients to the public as a whole. You have a responsibility to uphold the ethical standards of your profession and to advocate for policies that protect the health and well-being of the public.

Chapter 14: Continuing Education and Certification

Aromatherapy Training and Certification

The Cornerstones of Aromatherapy Training: A Holistic Approach

A comprehensive aromatherapy training program encompasses a diverse range of subjects, laying the groundwork for a profound understanding of the field. Botany, the study of plants, provides insights into the origin and properties of essential oils, while chemistry unravels their molecular composition and therapeutic actions. Anatomy and physiology illuminate the intricate workings of the human body, enabling practitioners to tailor aromatherapy treatments to individual needs.

The core of aromatherapy training lies in the sensory exploration of essential oils. Through olfactory experiences and hands-on workshops, students develop a refined sense of smell and learn to discern the subtle nuances of different scents. They delve into the therapeutic properties of essential oils, exploring their emotional, physical, and energetic effects.

The Art of Aromatherapy Application: A Journey of Healing and Transformation

Armed with a solid theoretical foundation, aromatherapy students embark on the practical application of essential oils. They learn various techniques to incorporate scents into daily routines, including inhalation, topical application, and diffusion. In-depth instruction covers massage, reflexology, and other complementary therapies, empowering practitioners to create personalized treatments that address specific health concerns and promote relaxation.

The therapeutic benefits of aromatherapy are vast and multifaceted. Essential oils have been shown to alleviate stress, anxiety, and depression; enhance sleep quality; boost immunity; and provide relief from a range of physical ailments, including pain, headaches, and respiratory issues. By understanding the therapeutic properties of individual oils and the art of blending, practitioners can create bespoke treatments that cater to each client's unique needs.

Certification: The Hallmark of Professionalism and Expertise

Upon completion of a comprehensive aromatherapy training program, students may pursue certification. Certification validates a practitioner's knowledge and skills, demonstrating their commitment to providing safe and effective aromatherapy treatments. Various organizations offer certification programs, each with its own set of requirements and standards.

Choosing the Right Aromatherapy Training Program: A Path to Excellence

Navigating the landscape of aromatherapy training programs can be daunting, but careful consideration of a few key factors can guide you towards the right choice. Look for programs that are accredited by reputable organizations, ensuring that they meet industry standards. Consider the duration and intensity of the program, ensuring that it aligns with your learning goals and time constraints.

Instructors play a vital role in the learning experience. Seek programs led by experienced aromatherapists with a passion for sharing their knowledge. Their guidance and expertise will prove invaluable in shaping your understanding and skills.

The Future of Aromatherapy: A Tapestry of Innovation and Growth

The future of aromatherapy is as fragrant and alluring as the essential oils themselves. Advances in research are continuously expanding our knowledge of the therapeutic benefits of essential oils, leading to the development of new applications and treatment protocols.

A growing appreciation for holistic and complementary

therapies is driving the demand for skilled aromatherapy practitioners. As more individuals seek natural solutions for health and well-being, aromatherapy is poised to play an increasingly significant role in the healthcare landscape. Through comprehensive training and certification, practitioners gain the knowledge and skills to harness the power of essential oils, empowering them to create personalized treatments that address the unique needs of each individual. As the future of aromatherapy unfolds, its potential for innovation and growth remains as limitless as the fragrant embrace it offers.

Professional Development for Aromatherapists

CPD for aromatherapists encompasses a range of activities designed to enhance their knowledge, skills, and competencies. This pursuit fosters not only personal growth but also elevates the overall standards of the profession. Aromatherapists engaged in CPD demonstrate a commitment to delivering safe, evidence-based, and client-centered care.

Key Areas of Professional Development for Aromatherapists

The scope of professional development for aromatherapists encompasses a diverse array of subjects, including:

- Botanical and Chemical Expertise: Aromatherapists must possess a deep understanding of the botanical origins, chemical compositions, and therapeutic properties of essential oils. CPD courses in these areas enhance their ability to select and blend oils effectively for specific client needs.

- Safety and Pharmacology: Ensuring the safe and responsible use of essential oils is a fundamental aspect of aromatherapy practice. CPD programs in safety and pharmacology equip aromatherapists with the knowledge to identify potential contraindications, interactions, and adverse effects.

- Clinical Applications: Aromatherapy finds application in various health and wellness settings, including stress management, pain relief, skin care, and emotional well-being. CPD courses in clinical applications empower aromatherapists to tailor their treatments to diverse client populations.

- Ethical and Legal Considerations: Aromatherapists are bound by ethical and legal obligations. CPD programs in these areas ensure their awareness of industry regulations, privacy laws, and informed consent procedures.

- Business Management and Marketing: For aromatherapists operating as independent practitioners, CPD in business management and marketing can enhance their entrepreneurial skills. This includes developing business plans, marketing strategies, and client relationship management.

Benefits of Professional Development for Aromatherapists

Embracing professional development offers numerous benefits to aromatherapists:

- Enhanced Knowledge and Skills: CPD enables aromatherapists to stay abreast of the latest research and best practices in the field. This expanded knowledge base empowers them to provide more effective and comprehensive treatments.

- Increased Confidence and Credibility: Participation in CPD demonstrates a commitment to ongoing learning and professional growth. This enhances an aromatherapist's confidence in their abilities and bolsters their credibility in the eyes of clients and colleagues.

- Professional Recognition: Many professional organizations and regulatory bodies require aromatherapists to engage in CPD to maintain their credentials. This recognition underscores the importance of ongoing education in the field.

- Personal Fulfillment: CPD fosters personal growth and intellectual stimulation. By continuously expanding their knowledge and skills, aromatherapists cultivate a sense of accomplishment and purpose.

Professional development is an essential cornerstone of aromatherapist practice. By actively engaging in CPD activities, aromatherapists can refine their knowledge, enhance their skills, and stay abreast of evolving best practices. This unwavering commitment to learning ensures that they remain at the forefront of their profession, delivering safe, effective, and client-centered care that empowers individuals to achieve optimal well-being.

Chapter 15: Research and Evidence

Clinical Studies on Aromatherapy

Efficacy of Aromatherapy in Pain Management

Numerous clinical trials have investigated the analgesic effects of aromatherapy in managing pain. A meta-analysis of 15 studies found that lavender oil, when inhaled or topically applied, significantly reduced pain intensity in various conditions, including postoperative pain, labor pain, and headaches. Another study demonstrated the effectiveness of peppermint oil in alleviating tension headaches, with a 50% reduction in pain severity within 15 minutes of inhalation.

Aromatherapy's Role in Reducing Anxiety and Depression

Clinical studies have also explored the anxiolytic and antidepressant effects of aromatherapy. A randomized controlled trial found that inhaling a blend of lavender and orange essential oils for 15 minutes significantly reduced anxiety levels in individuals with generalized anxiety disorder. Additionally, a systematic review of 12 studies reported that lavender oil was effective in reducing symptoms of postpartum depression, with improvements in mood and sleep quality.

Effects on Sleep and Cognitive Function

Aromatherapy has shown promising results in improving sleep quality and cognitive function. A study involving older adults with sleep disturbances found that inhaling lavender oil before bedtime significantly enhanced sleep duration and quality. Another clinical trial demonstrated that rosemary oil inhalation improved cognitive performance in healthy individuals, particularly in tasks involving memory and attention.

Physiological Effects of Aromatherapy

Clinical studies have also investigated the physiological effects of aromatherapy. A study examining the impact of lavender oil on blood pressure and heart rate found that inhalation of the oil led to significant reductions in both parameters, suggesting its potential in managing stress-related cardiovascular conditions. Additionally, a trial on the topical application of peppermint oil showed that it stimulated the cutaneous microcirculation, potentially improving blood flow to local tissues.

Safety and Tolerability

While aromatherapy is generally considered safe, it is important to note that certain essential oils may cause adverse effects, particularly in high doses or when ingested. Clinical studies have reported cases of contact dermatitis, allergic reactions, and gastrointestinal upset associated with the use of some oils. Therefore, it is crucial to consult with a qualified healthcare professional before using essential oils for therapeutic purposes.

Limitations of Clinical Studies on Aromatherapy

Despite the growing body of research, there are certain limitations to clinical studies on aromatherapy that should be considered. Some studies have small sample sizes or lack rigorous methodology, potentially limiting the generalizability of the findings. Additionally, the subjective nature of many aromatherapy outcomes, such as pain and mood, can introduce bias into study results.

Clinical studies provide valuable insights into the potential benefits and limitations of aromatherapy. While there is promising evidence supporting its efficacy in managing pain, anxiety, depression, and sleep disturbances, further research is needed to establish clear dosage guidelines, identify optimal essential oil combinations, and fully understand the mechanisms of action. It is essential to approach aromatherapy with caution and consult with qualified healthcare professionals to ensure safe and effective use.

Efficacy of Essential Oils

Mode of Action

Essential oils exert their effects through various

mechanisms, including:

Antimicrobial activity: Many essential oils contain compounds that inhibit the growth of bacteria, fungi, and viruses. This property makes them potentially useful for treating infections and preventing their spread.
Anti-inflammatory effects: Some essential oils, such as lavender and chamomile, have been shown to reduce inflammation, which can be beneficial for conditions like arthritis and skin irritation.
Sedative and calming effects: Certain essential oils, such as lavender and bergamot, have calming and sedative properties that can help promote relaxation and sleep.
Stimulating and energizing effects: Other essential oils, such as peppermint and rosemary, have stimulating effects that can improve alertness and energy levels.

Evidence of Efficacy

Numerous studies have investigated the efficacy of essential oils for various applications. Here are some examples:

Lavender oil for anxiety and sleep: A meta-analysis of 15 studies found that lavender oil significantly reduced anxiety symptoms and improved sleep quality.
Tea tree oil for acne: Tea tree oil has been shown to be effective in reducing acne lesions and improving skin health.
Eucalyptus oil for respiratory infections: Eucalyptus oil has expectorant and decongestant properties, making it useful for treating respiratory infections like colds and flu.
Peppermint oil for headaches: Peppermint oil applied

topically has been found to relieve tension headaches.

Limitations and Cautions

While essential oils can be beneficial in certain applications, it is important to note their limitations and potential risks:

Limited research: While some essential oils have been studied extensively, the research on many others is limited. More studies are needed to fully understand their efficacy and safety.
Potential for interactions: Essential oils can interact with certain medications, so it is crucial to consult with a healthcare professional before using them if you are taking any prescription drugs.
Skin irritation: Some essential oils can be irritating to the skin, especially if applied undiluted. Always dilute essential oils in a carrier oil, such as jojoba or almond oil, before applying them to the skin.
Potential toxicity: Some essential oils, such as pennyroyal and thuja, are toxic and should never be used.

Essential oils can be a valuable addition to your health and wellness routine, but it is essential to approach their use with caution and to have realistic expectations. While they may be effective for certain applications, they are not a substitute for conventional medical care. Always consult with a qualified healthcare professional before using essential oils, especially if you have any underlying health conditions or are taking any medications.

Aromatherapy in Integrative Medicine

Essential Oils: Nature's Aromatic Arsenal

At the heart of aromatherapy lies the utilization of essential oils, highly concentrated liquids that capture the therapeutic properties of aromatic plants. These volatile compounds, extracted through methods such as steam distillation, cold pressing, or solvent extraction, possess a vast array of pharmacological activities, including antimicrobial, analgesic, anti-inflammatory, and anxiolytic effects.

Mechanisms of Action: A Journey Through the Senses

The therapeutic effects of aromatherapy are mediated through various physiological and psychological pathways. When inhaled, aromatic molecules travel directly to the olfactory bulb, triggering neural responses that impact the limbic system, a brain region associated with emotions, memories, and behavior. Additionally, essential oils can be absorbed through the skin, where they interact with receptors and enzymes to exert their therapeutic effects.

Evidence-Based Applications: Embracing Aromatherapy's Therapeutic Scope

Numerous scientific studies have explored the therapeutic potential of aromatherapy in various healthcare settings. In the realm of pain management, lavender oil has demonstrated efficacy in reducing postoperative pain and nausea. Peppermint oil, renowned for its invigorating properties, has been shown to enhance cognitive function and reduce fatigue in patients with chronic conditions.

Aromatherapy has also found a place in the management of stress and anxiety. Studies have indicated that the calming aroma of chamomile oil can effectively reduce anxiety levels and promote relaxation. Similarly, bergamot oil has been found to possess antidepressant properties, offering hope to individuals struggling with mood disorders.

Integrating Aromatherapy into Clinical Practice: A Collaborative Approach

The integration of aromatherapy into clinical practice requires a collaborative approach between healthcare professionals and patients. Practitioners should possess a thorough understanding of essential oils' properties, contraindications, and potential interactions with medications. Patients, in turn, should be actively involved in the selection of scents and application methods that resonate with their individual needs and preferences.

Empowering Patients: Self-Care Strategies for Holistic Well-being

Beyond clinical settings, aromatherapy empowers individuals to take charge of their well-being through self-care practices. Diffusing essential oils in the home or workplace can create a relaxing or invigorating atmosphere. Adding a few drops of lavender oil to a warm bath can promote restful sleep. Topical application of essential oils, diluted in a carrier oil, can provide localized pain relief or enhance skin health.

Ethical Considerations: Ensuring Safe and Responsible Use

While aromatherapy offers numerous therapeutic benefits, it is essential to emphasize ethical considerations to ensure safe and responsible use. Essential oils should never be ingested or applied undiluted to the skin. Pregnant women and individuals with certain medical conditions should consult with a healthcare professional before using aromatherapy. By embracing the therapeutic potential of aromatic compounds and integrating them into personalized care plans, healthcare practitioners and patients alike can unlock a holistic and empowering approach to well-being. As research continues to unravel the complexities of essential oils, aromatherapy promises to play an increasingly significant role in integrative medicine, offering a gentle yet powerful means to promote physical, emotional, and spiritual health.

Chapter 16: Quality and Regulation

Essential Oil Quality Standards

Defining Essential Oil Quality

Essential oil quality is determined by a combination of factors, including:

Plant species and cultivar: The specific plant species and cultivar used for extraction influence the composition and properties of the oil.
Extraction method: Different extraction methods, such as steam distillation, cold pressing, and solvent extraction, can affect the yield and quality of the oil.
Growing conditions: Environmental factors, such as soil composition, climate, and altitude, impact the plant's growth and the quality of its essential oils.
Harvesting time: The time of year and the plant's maturity at harvest influence the concentration and composition of the oil.
Storage conditions: Proper storage practices, such as cool temperatures and protection from light, are essential to maintain the oil's quality over time.

Importance of Quality Standards

Establishing and adhering to essential oil quality standards is crucial for several reasons:

Purity: High-quality standards ensure that essential oils are free from adulterants, such as synthetic fragrances, fillers, or carrier oils. Purity is essential for therapeutic efficacy and safety.
Authenticity: Quality standards verify that the essential oil is derived from the specified plant species and is not a blend or counterfeit. This ensures that consumers are getting what they pay for.
Safety: Adulterated or low-quality essential oils may contain harmful chemicals or contaminants that can cause adverse health effects, such as skin irritation or respiratory problems.
Therapeutic efficacy: High-quality essential oils contain the optimal concentration of active compounds, ensuring their therapeutic benefits.

International Standards

Several international organizations have established standards for essential oil quality, including:

International Organization for Standardization (ISO): ISO 3528 provides guidelines for the sampling, testing, and evaluation of essential oils.
European Pharmacopoeia (Ph. Eur.): Ph. Eur. monographs establish quality specifications for essential oils used in medicinal products.

United States Pharmacopeia (USP): USP provides monographs and testing methods for essential oils used in pharmaceutical applications.

Testing and Verification

To ensure compliance with quality standards, essential oils undergo rigorous testing, including:

Gas chromatography-mass spectrometry (GC-MS): This technique identifies and quantifies the chemical components of the oil, verifying its composition and purity.
Optical rotation: This test measures the rotation of plane-polarized light passing through the oil, providing information about its structural integrity.
Refractive index: The refractive index of an oil is a measure of its light-bending properties, indicating its chemical composition and quality.
Specific gravity: This test determines the density of the oil, which is characteristic of the specific plant species.

Consumer Awareness and Responsibility

Consumers play a vital role in ensuring essential oil quality by:

Purchasing from reputable sources: Look for companies that follow established quality standards and provide third-party verification.
Reading product labels carefully: Verify the botanical name of the plant, the extraction method, and any other relevant information.
Storing essential oils properly: Follow storage guidelines to

maintain the oil's integrity and prevent degradation. Using essential oils safely: Consult with a healthcare professional or qualified aromatherapist for guidance on proper dilution and application methods.

Essential oil quality standards are essential for ensuring the purity, authenticity, safety, and therapeutic efficacy of these natural extracts. By adhering to established standards and conducting rigorous testing, reputable essential oil companies provide consumers with the highest quality oils, enabling them to reap the full benefits of these natural remedies. Informed consumers who purchase from trusted sources and use essential oils safely can experience the transformative power of these aromatic treasures.

Regulatory Considerations for Aromatherapy Products

Global Regulatory Framework

The regulation of aromatherapy products varies significantly across jurisdictions. While some countries have established comprehensive regulatory frameworks, others have yet to implement specific regulations. However, certain overarching principles guide the global approach to aromatherapy product regulation:

Product Safety: Regulations focus on ensuring the safety of aromatherapy products for consumers, minimizing the risk of adverse reactions or harmful effects.

Ingredient Disclosure: Consumers have the right to know the ingredients in aromatherapy products to make informed choices about their use.

Accurate Labeling: Product labels must provide clear and accurate information about the contents, usage instructions, and any potential risks or precautions.

Quality Control: Manufacturers must implement quality control measures to ensure the consistency and purity of their products.

Specific Regulations by Region

Europe:

The European Union (EU) has established a robust regulatory framework for aromatherapy products under the Cosmetic Products Regulation (EC) No. 1223. 2009. Key provisions include:

All cosmetic products, including aromatherapy products, must undergo a safety assessment by a qualified expert before being placed on the market.

Restricted and prohibited substances are listed in Annexes II and III of the Regulation.

Product labels must include a list of ingredients, contact information for the responsible person, and any necessary warnings or precautions.

United States:

In the United States, the Food and Drug Administration (FDA) regulates aromatherapy products differently depending on their intended use:

Cosmetics: Aromatherapy products intended for topical application and cosmetic purposes are regulated as cosmetics. The FDA has not established specific regulations for aromatherapy cosmetics, but manufacturers must comply with general cosmetic safety requirements.
Drugs: Aromatherapy products marketed with therapeutic claims are considered drugs and must undergo FDA approval before being sold.
Dietary Supplements: Some aromatherapy products are sold as dietary supplements, and the FDA regulates their safety and labeling under the Dietary Supplement Health and Education Act (DSHEA).

Other Regions:

Regulations for aromatherapy products in other regions vary widely. Some countries, such as Australia and Canada, have adopted similar approaches to the EU, while others have less stringent or specific regulations.

Considerations for Manufacturers

Manufacturers of aromatherapy products have several key responsibilities under regulatory frameworks:

Ingredient Sourcing: Obtain essential oils from reputable suppliers who can provide certificates of analysis and ensure quality and purity.
Product Safety Assessment: Conduct thorough safety assessments to evaluate the potential risks and benefits of their products.

Labeling Compliance: Ensure product labels are accurate, compliant with regulations, and provide all necessary information for consumers.

Quality Control: Implement quality control measures throughout the production process to maintain product consistency and purity.

Recordkeeping: Maintain detailed records of all safety assessments, ingredient sourcing, and production processes for regulatory inspection.

Considerations for Distributors and Consumers

Distributors and consumers also play important roles in ensuring the safety and efficacy of aromatherapy products:

Distributor Responsibilities: Distributors should ensure they are sourcing products from reputable manufacturers and that products are properly labeled and meet regulatory requirements.

Consumer Education: Consumers should educate themselves about the potential benefits and risks of aromatherapy, research products carefully, and only purchase from trusted sources.

Safe Usage: Follow usage instructions carefully, avoid ingesting or applying essential oils directly to sensitive areas, and seek professional guidance if necessary.

Regulatory considerations are essential for the safe and responsible use of aromatherapy products. Manufacturers, distributors, and consumers must be aware of the regulations applicable to their jurisdiction and take steps to comply with these requirements. By adhering to regulatory standards, ensuring product safety, and promoting informed consumer choice, we can harness the benefits of aromatherapy while minimizing potential risks.

Chapter 17: Plant Profiles

Botanical Descriptions and Properties of Key Essential Oils

Botanical Descriptions

Lavender (Lavandula angustifolia): Lavender is a small, flowering shrub native to the Mediterranean region. It is characterized by its purple flowers and sweet, floral scent. Lavender essential oil is known for its calming and relaxing effects, making it a popular choice for sleep and stress relief.

Peppermint (Mentha piperita): Peppermint is a hybrid mint plant known for its strong, minty aroma. It is native to Europe and North America and is widely cultivated for its essential oil. Peppermint essential oil is known for its stimulating and invigorating effects, making it a popular choice for boosting energy and focus.

Tea Tree (Melaleuca alternifolia): Tea tree is a small tree native to Australia. It is known for its potent antiseptic and antimicrobial properties. Tea tree essential oil is often used to treat skin infections, acne, and other skin conditions.

Eucalyptus (Eucalyptus globulus): Eucalyptus is a tall, evergreen tree native to Australia. It is known for its strong, camphoraceous scent. Eucalyptus essential oil is known for its expectorant and decongestant properties, making it a popular choice for treating respiratory infections.

Frankincense (Boswellia serrata): Frankincense is a small tree native to the Middle East and North Africa. It is known for its rich, balsamic scent. Frankincense essential oil has been used for centuries for its anti-inflammatory and pain-relieving properties.

Chemical Composition and Properties

Essential oils are complex mixtures of hundreds of different chemical compounds. These compounds can vary depending on the plant species, growing conditions, and extraction method. Some of the key chemical constituents of essential oils include:

Terpenes: Terpenes are the most common compounds found in essential oils. They are responsible for the characteristic scents of many plants. Some common terpenes include limonene, pinene, and myrcene.
Esters: Esters are known for their sweet, fruity aromas. Some common esters include linalyl acetate, geranyl acetate, and bergamotyl acetate.
Aldehydes: Aldehydes are known for their strong, spicy scents. Some common aldehydes include cinnamaldehyde, citral, and vanillin.
Phenols: Phenols are known for their antiseptic and

antimicrobial properties. Some common phenols include thymol, carvacrol, and eugenol.

The chemical composition of an essential oil determines its therapeutic properties. For example, lavender essential oil is rich in linalyl acetate, which is known for its calming effects, while peppermint essential oil is rich in menthol, which is known for its stimulating effects.

Therapeutic Uses

Essential oils have a wide range of therapeutic uses, including:

Stress relief: Essential oils such as lavender, chamomile, and bergamot can help to reduce stress and anxiety.
Pain relief: Essential oils such as frankincense, myrrh, and rosemary can help to relieve pain and inflammation.
Sleep improvement: Essential oils such as lavender, valerian root, and chamomile can help to promote relaxation and sleep.
Respiratory health: Essential oils such as eucalyptus, peppermint, and tea tree can help to clear congestion and support respiratory health.
Skin care: Essential oils such as tea tree, lavender, and frankincense can help to improve skin health and treat various skin conditions.

Safety Considerations

Essential oils are generally safe when used properly. However, some precautions should be taken to ensure their safe use:

Do not ingest essential oils orally.
Dilute essential oils with a carrier oil before applying them to the skin.
Avoid using essential oils on children or pregnant women.
If you have any underlying health conditions, consult with a healthcare professional before using essential oils.

Essential oils are powerful natural remedies that can offer a wide range of therapeutic benefits. By understanding the botanical descriptions and properties of key essential oils, you can safely and effectively use them to support your health and well-being.

Therapeutic Applications and Safety Guidelines

Musculoskeletal Conditions: Bowen therapy effectively relieves pain and stiffness associated with musculoskeletal conditions such as back pain, neck pain, frozen shoulder, tennis elbow, carpal tunnel syndrome, and plantar fasciitis. By releasing fascial restrictions and promoting muscle relaxation, Bowen therapy alleviates discomfort and improves mobility.

Neurological Conditions: Bowen therapy has shown promise in improving symptoms of neurological conditions, including migraines, headaches, multiple sclerosis, Parkinson's disease, and autism spectrum disorder. The gentle movements stimulate the nervous system, promoting relaxation and reducing sensory overload, which can alleviate pain, improve balance, and enhance cognitive function.

Physiological Conditions: Bowen therapy supports various physiological processes, including digestion, circulation, and immune function. By addressing fascial adhesions and promoting lymphatic drainage, Bowen therapy improves digestion, reduces inflammation, and boosts the body's ability to fight off infection.

Safety Guidelines for Bowen Therapy

Bowen therapy is generally considered safe when performed by a qualified practitioner. However, as with any manual therapy, there are certain precautions to be aware of.

Pre-Treatment Considerations: Individuals with acute injuries, severe medical conditions, or recent surgery should consult a healthcare professional before receiving Bowen therapy. Pregnant women should also consult their healthcare provider to determine if Bowen therapy is appropriate.

During Treatment: Bowen therapists apply gentle pressure during the treatment. If you experience any discomfort or pain, inform the therapist immediately. They will adjust the pressure or modify the technique to ensure your comfort.

Post-Treatment Care: After a Bowen therapy session, you may experience mild fatigue or soreness for a few days. Rest, hydration, and light activity are recommended to facilitate the body's healing response. Avoid strenuous exercise or heavy lifting immediately after treatment.

Contraindications: Bowen therapy is not recommended for individuals with certain conditions, such as deep vein thrombosis, severe osteoporosis, or open wounds. Pregnant women in their first trimester should also avoid Bowen therapy.

Finding a Qualified Bowen Therapist

To ensure the safety and effectiveness of Bowen therapy, it is crucial to find a qualified practitioner. Look for practitioners who:

Are certified by a reputable Bowen therapy organization.
Have received comprehensive training and hold professional liability insurance.
Maintain a clean and professional work environment.
Are attentive to your concerns and provide clear instructions before and after treatment.

By adhering to these safety guidelines and choosing a qualified practitioner, you can enjoy the therapeutic benefits of Bowen therapy while minimizing any potential risks.

Chapter 18: Blending Formulations

Step-by-Step Guide to Blending Essential Oils

Essential oils possess an array of therapeutic benefits, ranging from promoting relaxation and alleviating stress to boosting immunity and enhancing cognitive function. However, due to their potency, it is essential to dilute them with a carrier oil, such as jojoba, almond, or coconut oil, before applying them to the skin or inhaling them. This dilution ensures safe and effective use, preventing potential skin irritation or other adverse reactions.

Step 2: Choosing the Right Essential Oils

The art of blending essential oils lies in selecting the perfect combination of scents and therapeutic properties to achieve a desired outcome. Whether you seek relaxation, invigoration, or a specific therapeutic benefit, there is an essential oil blend waiting to fulfill your needs.

For a calming and relaxing blend, consider combining lavender, chamomile, and bergamot oils. These oils possess sedative and anxiolytic properties, making them ideal for unwinding after a long day or promoting restful sleep. In contrast, if you desire an invigorating blend to boost your energy and focus, try combining rosemary, peppermint, and grapefruit oils. These oils are known for their stimulating and uplifting effects, helping you to stay alert and productive.

If you have a specific therapeutic goal in mind, such as alleviating headaches or improving digestion, research the individual essential oils that have been shown to address those ailments. For instance, peppermint oil is commonly used for headache relief, while ginger oil is known to aid digestion. By combining these oils with other complementary scents, you can create a tailored blend that targets your specific needs.

Step 3: Determining the Correct Dilution Ratio

Once you have chosen your essential oils, it is essential to determine the appropriate dilution ratio for your intended use. The dilution ratio refers to the proportion of essential oils to carrier oil. The ideal ratio depends on several factors, including the potency of the essential oils, the desired strength of the blend, and the method of application.

For topical applications, such as massage or skincare, a dilution ratio of 2-3% is generally recommended. This means adding 2-3 drops of essential oils to every 10ml of carrier oil. For inhalation, a lower dilution ratio of 1-2% is suitable, as the essential oils will be more concentrated when diffused into the air.

It is important to note that some essential oils, such as cinnamon and oregano, are highly concentrated and should be used with caution. Always refer to the safety guidelines provided by the essential oil manufacturer to ensure proper dilution and avoid any potential risks.

Step 4: Blending the Essential Oils

Now comes the exciting part - blending your chosen essential oils. To ensure an even distribution and optimal therapeutic benefits, follow these steps:

- Gather a clean, dark-colored glass bottle or rollerball for storing your blend.
- Add the carrier oil to the bottle, filling it to the desired level.
- Using a dropper, carefully add the essential oils to the carrier oil, following the predetermined dilution ratio.
- Gently swirl the bottle to blend the oils thoroughly. Avoid shaking the bottle vigorously, as this can create air bubbles and alter the blend's consistency.

Step 5: Testing the Blend and Adjusting

Before using your newly created blend, it is advisable to test it on a small area of your skin to ensure there are no adverse reactions. Apply a dime-sized amount to the inner forearm and wait 24 hours to monitor for any irritation or discomfort. If no reaction occurs, you can proceed with using the blend as intended.

If the blend feels too strong or too weak, you can adjust

the dilution ratio accordingly. To make the blend stronger, add a few more drops of essential oils and swirl gently to combine. If the blend is too strong, add more carrier oil to dilute it further.

Step 6: Storing and Using Your Blend

Proper storage is crucial to preserve the integrity and shelf life of your essential oil blend. Store the blend in a cool, dark place away from direct sunlight and heat. Dark-colored glass bottles help protect the blend from degradation caused by light exposure.

When using your blend, follow the recommended dilution ratio and application method. For topical applications, massage the blend into the desired area using gentle circular motions. For inhalation, add a few drops to a diffuser or inhale directly from the bottle, taking deep, slow breaths.

Additional Tips for Blending Essential Oils:

- Start with a simple blend of 2-3 essential oils to develop your blending skills gradually.
- Experiment with different combinations of scents to find what appeals to you.
- Keep a notebook to record your blends and their effects for future reference.
- Seek guidance from a qualified aromatherapist if you have any specific health concerns or require personalized recommendations.

Blending essential oils is a captivating journey of self-discovery and holistic well-being. By understanding the basics, choosing the right oils, diluting them correctly, blending them harmoniously, and using them safely, you can harness the transformative power of essential oils to enhance your life in countless ways.

Blend Recipes for Common Ailments and Conditions

Choosing the Right Oils: A Guide to Essential Properties

Selecting the appropriate essential oils for your blend is crucial. Consider the therapeutic properties of each oil and its potential interactions with others. For example, lavender is renowned for its calming and relaxing effects, while peppermint invigorates and promotes mental clarity. Bergamot uplifts mood, and tea tree possesses antimicrobial properties. By carefully selecting oils with complementary or synergistic actions, you can create potent blends that effectively target specific health concerns.

Crafting Effective Blends: Achieving Balance and Harmony

The art of crafting effective blends lies in achieving a harmonious balance of scents and therapeutic properties. Start with a few drops of each chosen oil, gradually adjusting the proportions until you find a blend that resonates with you both aromatically and therapeutically. Experiment with different combinations to discover synergistic effects that meet your individual needs.

Blend Recipes for Common Ailments and Conditions

1. Stress and Anxiety Relief Blend:

Lavender (5 drops)
Bergamot (3 drops)
Frankincense (2 drops)

Inhale this blend from a diffuser or apply it topically to promote relaxation and reduce stress.

2. Headache Relief Blend:

Peppermint (4 drops)
Eucalyptus (3 drops)
Lavender (2 drops)

Apply this blend to your temples or inhale it from a tissue to alleviate headache pain and promote mental clarity.

3. Sleep Enhancement Blend:

Lavender (6 drops)
Roman chamomile (4 drops)
Ylang-ylang (2 drops)

Diffuse this blend in your bedroom or apply it to your pillowcase to promote restful sleep and reduce insomnia.

4. Respiratory Support Blend:

Eucalyptus (5 drops)
Peppermint (3 drops)

Tea tree (2 drops)

Add this blend to a diffuser or inhale it directly from a tissue to support respiratory health, clear congestion, and reduce inflammation.

5. Immune Boosting Blend:

Lemon (5 drops)
Tea tree (4 drops)
Rosemary (3 drops)

Diffuse this blend throughout your home or apply it topically to strengthen the immune system and protect against infection.

Safety Considerations for Aromatherapy Blends

Always dilute essential oils in a carrier oil, such as jojoba or coconut oil, before applying them to the skin.
Avoid using essential oils on children or pregnant women without consulting a healthcare professional.
Some essential oils may interact with certain medications. Consult with your doctor if you have any concerns.
Store essential oils in a cool, dark place to preserve their therapeutic properties.

Chapter 19: Resources

Aromatherapy Organizations and Associations

The field of aromatherapy has witnessed a surge in popularity in recent years, leading to the establishment of numerous organizations and associations dedicated to its advancement. These entities play a pivotal role in promoting the responsible use and dissemination of knowledge about aromatherapy, fostering professional development, and advocating for the rights and interests of practitioners.

Professional Organizations

1. National Association for Holistic Aromatherapy (NAHA)

Founded in 1990, NAHA is the largest professional organization for aromatherapists in the United States. It offers certification programs, educational resources, and a code of ethics to ensure the highest standards of practice. NAHA advocates for the safe and effective use of essential oils and promotes research to advance the field.

2. International Federation of Aromatherapists (IFA)

Established in 1987, IFA is an international organization with members from over 30 countries. It aims to foster excellence in aromatherapy practice, promote education and training, and provide support to aromatherapists worldwide. IFA sets standards for professional qualifications and offers a range of educational programs.

3. Alliance of International Aromatherapists (AIA)

AIA is a global organization dedicated to the advancement of clinical aromatherapy. It provides educational resources, hosts conferences, and advocates for the use of essential oils in healthcare settings. AIA also collaborates with other organizations to promote evidence-based aromatherapy practices.

4. National Association of Certified Clinical Aromatherapists (NACCA)

NACCA is a professional organization for certified clinical aromatherapists. It offers continuing education programs, supports research, and promotes the integration of aromatherapy into mainstream healthcare. NACCA advocates for the recognition and reimbursement of aromatherapy services.

5. American College of Healthcare Sciences (ACHS)

ACHS is a leading provider of holistic healthcare education, including aromatherapy programs. It offers certification courses, master's degrees, and continuing education workshops for aromatherapists and other healthcare professionals. ACHS also conducts research and disseminates knowledge to promote the advancement of aromatherapy.

Industry Associations

1. Essential Oil Association of Australia (EOAA)

EOAA is the peak industry body for essential oil producers, distillers, and suppliers in Australia. It promotes the sustainable production and use of essential oils, advocates for industry best practices, and supports research and education. EOAA also provides information to consumers about the safe and effective use of essential oils.

2. European Federation of Essential Oils (EFFEO)

EFFEO is an umbrella organization representing the essential oil industry in Europe. It advocates for the safe and responsible use of essential oils, promotes sustainable practices, and collaborates with regulatory authorities to ensure the quality and safety of essential oils. EFFEO also organizes conferences and provides educational resources to industry stakeholders.

3. Natural Products Association (NPA)

NPA is a trade association representing the natural products industry, including essential oils. It advocates for the responsible production, marketing, and use of natural products, promotes consumer education, and supports research. NPA also provides industry updates and resources to its members.

4. Aromatic Plant Producers Association (APPA)

APPA is an international organization representing producers and suppliers of aromatic plants and their essential oils. It promotes sustainable cultivation practices, facilitates trade, and advocates for the recognition and protection of aromatic plant resources. APPA also provides market information and resources to its members.

5. International Fragrance Association (IFRA)

IFRA is an industry association representing fragrance manufacturers, suppliers, and users. It establishes safety standards for fragrance ingredients, develops guidelines for the responsible use of fragrance, and conducts research on fragrance safety. IFRA also provides educational resources to consumers and professionals.

Aromatherapy organizations and associations play a vital role in the development and advancement of the field. These entities provide a forum for professionals to connect, share knowledge, and advocate for responsible practices. By promoting education, research, and collaboration, they ensure the continued growth and credibility of aromatherapy as a holistic healthcare modality.

Essential Oil Suppliers

Purity and Authenticity: The Cornerstones of Essential Oil Quality

Purity and authenticity are paramount considerations when selecting essential oils. Pure essential oils are those that have not been adulterated with other substances, such as synthetic fragrances, carriers, or diluents. Authentic essential oils, on the other hand, are true to their botanical source, meaning they have not been altered or blended with oils from different plants.

Key Factors to Evaluate When Choosing Suppliers

Numerous factors influence the quality of essential oils supplied by different vendors. Here are some crucial aspects to assess:

Extraction Method: The method used to extract essential oils from plant material greatly impacts their chemical composition and therapeutic value. Steam distillation, cold pressing, and solvent extraction are common techniques, each with its advantages and disadvantages.

Plant Source: The botanical species and the geographical location where the plant is grown can significantly affect the essential oil's properties. Essential oils derived from specific cultivars or regions may exhibit unique characteristics and therapeutic benefits.

Organic Certification: Organic certification ensures that the plants used in essential oil production have been grown without the use of synthetic pesticides or fertilizers. Organic essential oils are considered purer and more environmentally friendly.

第三方测试: Reputable suppliers often provide third-party

test results that verify the purity and authenticity of their essential oils. These tests can assess parameters such as chemical composition, heavy metal content, and microbiological contamination.

口碑: The experiences and reviews of other consumers can offer valuable insights into the reliability and quality of essential oil suppliers. Reading online reviews and testimonials can provide a sense of the supplier's customer service and commitment to transparency.

Ethical and Sustainable Considerations

In addition to purity and authenticity, ethical and sustainable practices are important considerations when sourcing essential oils. Look for suppliers who:

Prioritize Sustainable Harvesting: Sustainable harvesting practices ensure that essential oil production does not deplete or harm plant populations or their ecosystems.

Support Fair Trade: Fair trade practices guarantee fair compensation for farmers and workers involved in the essential oil supply chain.

Promote Environmental Responsibility: Responsible suppliers minimize their environmental footprint by using eco-friendly extraction and packaging methods.

Selecting the right essential oil supplier is essential for harnessing the full therapeutic potential and enjoyment of these aromatic wonders. By prioritizing purity, authenticity, ethical considerations, and sustainability, you can confidently choose suppliers who offer high-quality essential oils that meet your needs and support your well-being.

Books and Journals on Aromatherapy

Some of the most popular books on aromatherapy include:

Aromatherapy for Beginners by Valerie Ann Worwood: This book is a great introduction to aromatherapy, covering the basics of essential oils, their properties, and how to use them safely and effectively.

The Complete Guide to Aromatherapy by Salvatore Battaglia: This book is a comprehensive guide to aromatherapy, covering everything from the history and science of essential oils to their therapeutic uses.

Aromatherapy: The Essential Guide by Patricia Davis: This book is a practical guide to aromatherapy, providing step-by-step instructions on how to use essential oils for a variety of purposes.

The Healing Intelligence of Essential Oils by Kurt Schnaubelt: This book explores the scientific evidence behind the therapeutic benefits of essential oils, providing a deeper understanding of their healing properties.

Aromatherapy for the Soul by Valerie Ann Worwood: This book focuses on the emotional and spiritual benefits of aromatherapy, providing guidance on how to use essential oils to promote relaxation, balance, and well-being.

Journals on Aromatherapy

In addition to books, there are also a number of journals dedicated to aromatherapy. These journals publish original research, clinical studies, and case reports on the therapeutic uses of essential oils. They are an essential resource for aromatherapists who want to stay up-to-date on the latest developments in the field.

Some of the most popular journals on aromatherapy include:

The International Journal of Aromatherapy
The Journal of Essential Oil Research
Aromatherapy Today
The National Association for Holistic Aromatherapy Journal
The Alliance of International Aromatherapists Journal

These journals provide a wealth of information on the therapeutic uses of essential oils, including:

Clinical studies on the efficacy of essential oils for a variety of conditions, such as anxiety, depression, pain, and inflammation.
Research on the mechanisms of action of essential oils.
Case reports on the successful use of essential oils in clinical practice.
Reviews of the latest research on aromatherapy.

Books and journals on aromatherapy provide a valuable resource for both beginners and experienced aromatherapists alike. By reading these resources, you can gain a deeper understanding of the therapeutic benefits of essential oils and how to use them safely and effectively.

Chapter 20: Conclusion

The Future of Aromatherapy

Integration with Advanced Technologies

Technological advancements are revolutionizing the delivery and application of aromatherapy. Nebulizers, diffusers, and inhalers equipped with microchip technology offer precise control over the release and dispersal of essential oils, ensuring optimal absorption and therapeutic effects. Smart home devices, integrated with aromatherapy diffusers, enable remote control and scheduling, allowing users to create personalized aromatic environments tailored to their individual needs.

Moreover, the convergence of aromatherapy with virtual reality (VR) and augmented reality (AR) technologies has opened up exciting possibilities. VR environments infused with specific aromas can immerse users in multisensory experiences designed to promote relaxation, reduce stress, and enhance cognitive function. AR applications can provide interactive guides on the selection and use of essential oils, empowering individuals to harness the benefits of aromatherapy with confidence.

Precision and Personalized Treatments

Advancements in analytical techniques and artificial intelligence (AI) are enabling the development of personalized aromatherapy treatments. AI algorithms can analyze individual profiles, including genetics, medical history, and lifestyle factors, to generate tailored recommendations for essential oil blends that address specific health concerns. This precision approach enhances the efficacy of aromatherapy and minimizes potential adverse effects.

Furthermore, wearable devices such as smartwatches and fitness trackers can monitor physiological responses to aromatherapy. By tracking heart rate, skin temperature, and other biomarkers, these devices provide real-time feedback on the effectiveness of different essential oil combinations. This data-driven approach empowers individuals to optimize their aromatherapy experience and achieve desired outcomes.

Integration into Healthcare and Wellness Practices

Aromatherapy is increasingly gaining acceptance within healthcare and wellness sectors. Hospitals and clinics are exploring the use of essential oils to reduce stress and anxiety in patients undergoing medical procedures, improve sleep quality, and alleviate pain. Complementary and alternative medicine practitioners are incorporating aromatherapy into their treatment plans to enhance the overall well-being of their clients.

Wellness centers and spas are recognizing the therapeutic benefits of aromatherapy and offering a wide range of services that incorporate essential oils, such as massage, facials, and meditation. Essential oils are also being used in the development of natural skincare and cosmetic products, leveraging their antioxidant, anti-inflammatory, and antimicrobial properties to promote healthy and radiant skin.

Research and Innovation

Ongoing research continues to expand our understanding of the therapeutic potential of essential oils. Studies are investigating the efficacy of aromatherapy in addressing mental health conditions such as anxiety, depression, and post-traumatic stress disorder (PTSD). Researchers are also exploring the use of essential oils as adjuvants to conventional cancer treatments, with promising results in reducing side effects and improving quality of life.

The development of novel essential oil extraction techniques and the identification of new bioactive compounds are opening up avenues for innovation in the aromatherapy industry. Advanced extraction methods, such as supercritical fluid extraction and headspace analysis, allow for the isolation of highly concentrated and pure essential oils with enhanced therapeutic properties.

Expanding Applications

The future of aromatherapy extends beyond traditional therapeutic uses. Essential oils are gaining recognition in various industries, including:

Agriculture: As natural pest repellents and plant growth

enhancers, essential oils offer sustainable alternatives to synthetic chemicals.

Education: Aromatherapy in classrooms has been shown to improve focus, reduce hyperactivity, and promote a positive learning environment.

Automotive: Essential oils are being used in air fresheners and interior materials to create pleasant and invigorating atmospheres in vehicles.

Hospitality: Hotels and resorts are incorporating aromatherapy into their guest experiences, offering essential oil-infused amenities and spa treatments to enhance relaxation and well-being.

The future of aromatherapy is bright with immense potential for innovation and expanded applications. Technological advancements, personalized treatments, integration into healthcare and wellness practices, ongoing research, and novel applications will continue to drive the growth of this industry. As we delve deeper into the world of essential oils, we unlock a vast array of possibilities for enhancing physical, emotional, and mental well-being in the years to come.

The Importance of Evidence-Based Practice

The Benefits of Evidence-Based Practice

EBP offers numerous benefits for professionals and the

individuals they serve. Firstly, it promotes improved patient outcomes and quality of care. Research has consistently demonstrated that interventions based on sound evidence lead to better health outcomes, reduced healthcare costs, and increased patient satisfaction. By utilizing the latest research findings, professionals can optimize their practices and deliver more effective and targeted interventions.

Secondly, EBP enhances professional credibility and expertise. By staying abreast of the latest research and incorporating evidence into their practice, professionals demonstrate their commitment to providing the highest quality of care. This commitment fosters trust and respect among colleagues, patients, and the community.

Thirdly, EBP promotes continuous professional development and learning. It requires professionals to critically appraise research findings, evaluate their relevance to their practice, and incorporate new knowledge into their decision-making. This ongoing learning process fosters a culture of professional growth and ensures that practitioners remain equipped with the most current knowledge and skills.

The Components of Evidence-Based Practice

EBP involves a systematic and rigorous process that consists of five key components:

1. Asking a Focused Clinical Question: The first step involves clearly defining the patient's problem or issue and formulating a specific question that can be addressed by

research evidence.

2. Searching for the Best Available Evidence: Using a systematic approach, professionals search for relevant research studies in databases and other sources. They critically appraise the studies to determine their quality and relevance.

3. Appraising the Evidence: Professionals carefully evaluate the research evidence to assess its validity, reliability, and applicability to their specific patient or situation. They consider the study design, sample size, and potential biases.

4. Integrating the Evidence with Clinical Expertise and Patient Values: The evidence is then integrated with the professional's clinical expertise and the patient's values and preferences. This integration ensures that the intervention or treatment plan is tailored to the individual's needs and circumstances.

5. Evaluating the Outcome: All in all, professionals monitor the patient's progress and evaluate the effectiveness of the intervention. They may adjust the plan based on the patient's response and new evidence that emerges.

The Challenges of Evidence-Based Practice

While EBP offers significant benefits, there are certain challenges associated with its implementation. These challenges include:

1. Time Constraints: Incorporating EBP into a busy clinical

practice can be time-consuming, especially for practitioners with heavy patient loads.

2. Access to Evidence: Practitioners may face challenges in accessing high-quality research evidence, particularly in rapidly evolving fields where new knowledge is constantly emerging.

3. Research-Practice Gap: Bridging the gap between research findings and practical implementation can be difficult, as research studies may not always be directly applicable to individual patients or settings.

4. Individual Differences: Patients vary in their preferences, values, and health conditions. Tailoring interventions based on individual needs while adhering to evidence-based guidelines can be a complex task.

Overcoming Challenges and Promoting EBP

Despite these challenges, promoting EBP is essential for delivering high-quality healthcare. To overcome these barriers, healthcare systems and professional organizations can:

1. Provide Training and Support: Offer training programs and resources to help professionals develop the skills and knowledge required for EBP.

2. Facilitate Access to Evidence: Create centralized databases and knowledge repositories to make research evidence easily accessible to practitioners.

3. Foster Collaboration: Encourage collaboration between researchers and practitioners to bridge the research-practice gap and facilitate the translation of research findings into clinical practice.

4. Incorporate EBP into Professional Development: Integrate EBP into professional development programs and continuing education requirements to promote ongoing learning and commitment to evidence-based practices.

Evidence-based practice is a vital approach that enables professionals to make informed decisions, improve patient outcomes, and enhance professional credibility. By incorporating the best available research evidence into their practice, professionals can provide high-quality, patient-centered care that is supported by the latest scientific knowledge. Overcoming the challenges associated with EBP and promoting its widespread adoption is essential for the advancement of healthcare and the well-being of patients.

Aromatherapy as a Holistic Health Approach

Essential oils can also be applied to the skin, where they are absorbed into the bloodstream. This allows them to interact with our cells and tissues, providing a variety of therapeutic benefits. Essential oils have been shown to have antibacterial, antiviral, antifungal, and anti-inflammatory properties. They can also help to improve circulation, reduce pain, and promote relaxation.

Aromatherapy can be used to treat a wide range of conditions, including:

Stress and anxiety
Depression
Insomnia
Headaches and migraines
Muscle pain and spasms
Skin conditions
Respiratory problems
Digestive problems

Aromatherapy is a safe and effective way to improve your health and well-being. It is a gentle and non-invasive therapy that can be used in conjunction with other treatments. If you are new to aromatherapy, it is important to talk to a qualified aromatherapist before using essential oils.

How to Use Aromatherapy

There are many different ways to use aromatherapy. The most common methods include:

Inhalation: You can inhale essential oils directly from the bottle, or you can add a few drops to a diffuser or humidifier. Inhaling essential oils is a great way to improve your mood, energy levels, and overall sense of well-being.
Topical application: You can apply essential oils to your skin, either diluted in a carrier oil or undiluted. Topical application of essential oils is a great way to treat skin conditions, muscle pain, and headaches.
Bathing: You can add a few drops of essential oils to your

bathwater. This is a great way to relax and unwind at the end of the day.

Choosing Essential Oils

There are many different essential oils available, each with its own unique properties. When choosing essential oils, it is important to consider your individual needs and preferences. Some of the most popular essential oils for aromatherapy include:

Lavender: Lavender is a calming and relaxing oil that is great for reducing stress and anxiety.
Peppermint: Peppermint is an invigorating and stimulating oil that is great for improving energy levels and focus.
Eucalyptus: Eucalyptus is a decongestant and expectorant that is great for treating respiratory problems.
Tea tree: Tea tree is an antibacterial and antifungal oil that is great for treating skin conditions.
Frankincense: Frankincense is an anti-inflammatory and pain-relieving oil that is great for treating muscle pain and headaches.

Safety Precautions

Essential oils are highly concentrated and can be harmful if not used properly. It is important to follow these safety precautions when using essential oils:

Never ingest essential oils. Essential oils are not meant to be swallowed. If you ingest an essential oil, call the poison control center immediately.
Dilute essential oils before applying them to your skin.

Essential oils can be irritating to the skin, so it is important to dilute them in a carrier oil before applying them. A good rule of thumb is to add 2-3 drops of essential oil to 1 ounce of carrier oil.

Avoid using essential oils on children under the age of 6. Essential oils can be harmful to young children, so it is important to avoid using them on children under the age of 6.

Do not use essential oils if you are pregnant or breastfeeding. Essential oils can cross the placenta and enter breast milk, so it is important to avoid using them if you are pregnant or breastfeeding.

Store essential oils in a cool, dark place. Essential oils are volatile and can degrade quickly if they are exposed to heat or light. Store essential oils in a cool, dark place to preserve their potency.

Printed in Great Britain
by Amazon